Tipping the Scales
in Your Favor

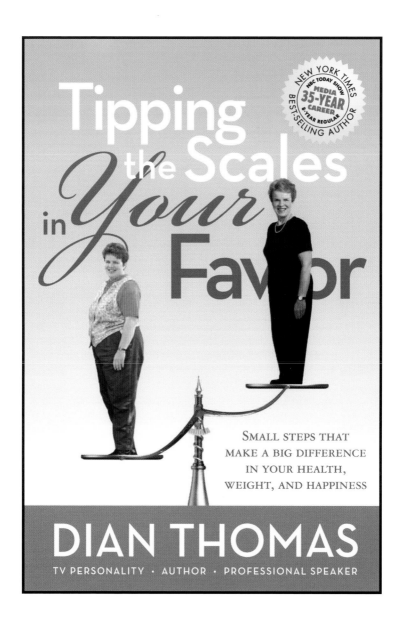

Tipping
the Scales
in *Your*
Fav☐r

NEW YORK TIMES
NBC TODAY SHOW
MEDIA
35-YEAR
CAREER
8-YEAR REGULAR
BEST-SELLING AUTHOR

SMALL STEPS THAT
MAKE A BIG DIFFERENCE
IN YOUR HEALTH,
WEIGHT, AND HAPPINESS

DIAN THOMAS
TV PERSONALITY · AUTHOR · PROFESSIONAL SPEAKER

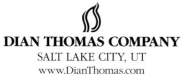

DIAN THOMAS COMPANY
SALT LAKE CITY, UT
www.DianThomas.com

Distributed by
Brigham Distribution
110 South 800 West
Brigham City, UT 84302-2400
(435) 723-6611

12 11 10 09 08 07 06 05 04 03

Library of Congress Control Number: 2011908114

Thomas, Dian
  Tipping the Scales in Your Favor: Small steps that will make a big difference in your health, weight, and happiness.

  Includes index
  ISBN 978-0-9621257-1-3
  1. Weight loss   2. Health   I. Title

NOTICE: The information in this book is true and complete to the best of my knowledge. All recommendations are made without guarantees on the part of the author/publisher. The author/publisher disclaims all liability in connection with the use of this information. A physical check-up is recommended.

For additional books by Dian Thomas, go to her Web site: www.DianThomas.com.

Back cover: Photo of Dian preparing to cook was taken by Stuart Johnson, *Deseret News.*

Dedication

This book is dedicated to Jackie Keller (photo, page 12). She kindled the spark that helped me realize I could lose weight. Her wisdom and support—and the accountability she required of me—led me to a healthier lifestyle.

Thank you, Jackie, for reaching out to me so that I could create a new life, unloading the burden of weight that has held me down for over fifteen years. With your wonderful assistance and insights, I won the losing game.

About Jackie Keller

Jackie's father passed away from a heart attack when she was just a teenager. She has made it her mission to help people live longer and healthier lives. "I have a personal commitment to help people circumvent heart disease and other chronic ailments," she explains. "It drives almost everything I do. It is my passion."

Jackie is the founding director of NutriFit™ LLC. She's a certified professional wellness coach, executive chef, and health educator. NutriFit's goal is to promote long-term health by providing full-service nutritional support and fresh gourmet meals to individuals and families nationwide.

Jackie holds a bachelor of science degree from the University of Southern California, and she received her culinary training from Le Cordon Bleu in Paris, France, and her coach training from Well-coaches International.

Jackie and her husband, Phil, are the parents of two children.

For more information on Jackie's wellness coaching and programs, go to www.jackiekeller.com or www.nutrifitonline.com/, or call 310-473-1989.

Acknowledgments

To create a product that I can be proud to put my name on, it took a cast of characters working behind the scenes. Each played a significant role in helping me produce this book. Thank you for your special support and help.

Jackie Keller approached me a few years ago and planted the seed that I could lose weight and worked with me step by step through the challenging and rewarding process. I have a new life now, and I love it.

Brian Mullahy first featured my story on Salt Lake City's KUTV Channel 2 Ten O'Clock News. Thank you for sharing my story.

Angie Hutchinson, lifestyle editor at the *Deseret News*, saw the KUTV broadcast and asked Valerie Phillips, their food editor, to write a feature story on my weight loss, which led to a bimonthly column and blog.

Dianne King, an editor with 30-plus years in the industry, took my words and polished them so they are concise, interesting, and to the point.

Supporting Editors: Valerie Phillips, Janet Stock, and Karen Christofferson also contributed their insights, wisdom, and blessings.

Richard Haight morphed the 50,000-plus words into a visual work of art.

Kent Merrell of Merrell Remington gave freely of his expertise and creativity in moving this project to completion.

Noel Hilden took many of the photos and also gave valuable support and ideas.

There were a score who read the copy and gave creative suggestions for organizing and polishing the material. Thank you to Marquette and Bill Mansell, Boyd Tuttle, Adriana Garcia, Shawn Bucher, Barbara Dahl, Dorothy De Mare, Cheri Thomas, Marla Jensen, Dr. Von Johnson, Todd Curtis, Carolyn Mosier, Dr. Phil Allsen, Colleen Peterson, and Debbie Evans.

Table of Contents

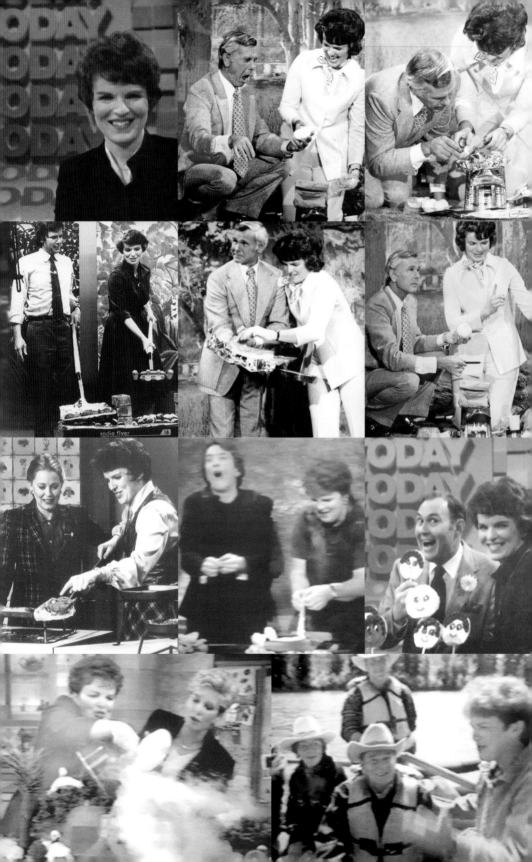

Chapter 1
Winning at the Losing Game

Many people remember me from my New York Times best-selling *Roughing It Easy* books and as a regular on NBC's *Today* show. For years, I was known as "MacGyver in a Skirt." I shared clever, creative, unique, and inexpensive ideas suitable for friends and family to enjoy while creating long-lasting memories.

Now that I have lost 125 pounds, I want to tell you how I gained the weight and what I eventually did about it. It is my desire to encourage others in their weight-loss quests. For me, fewer pounds meant a better life of more activity, more self-confidence, and more opportunities to experience travel and the fun things of life.

In 2003, at 5 feet 8 inches, I topped the scales at 326½ pounds, quite a jump from the 170 pounds I weighed in 1975 when I first appeared on NBC's *Tonight* show with Johnny Carson to demonstrate ideas from my first book, *Roughing It Easy*. My knees hurt so much that I began using a walker to help me get around the house. I once broke a friend's chair by sitting in it. If I ever got down on the floor, it was next to impossible to get back up. Fitting into a regular airplane seat was also a huge challenge.

Today, my weight hovers around 200 pounds, with just 10 to 20 more to go to reach my goal. Now I move like I'm young again! I can bike for miles at a time; last summer I completed a 480-mile bike expedition across the state of Iowa in a week. In one day I was even able to ride 100 miles, which I had never dreamed would be possible. I love walking, riding my bike, and doing water aerobics—and, yes, I have to push myself a bit to lift weights, but I know it is important to my health and I do it.

Instead of a gastric bypass or a quick-fix diet, I took a slow, methodical approach to weight change by adopting new habits. Through this process I average a half-pound to a pound a week. Even though it has been a slow go, all these single pounds have added up, and the weight has stayed off. The most difficult time for me is when I travel or eat at a friend's home. Although it's taken several years, my weight is under control, and I have regained my health. That's what I care about!

What I have learned is it's not the speed that counts, but the direction you're going. I do not call it a diet—I call it a lifestyle change.

Instead of one magic bullet, there are a number of steps to consistently follow, including keeping motivated, planning, eating right, exercising, and being accountable. It's like a symphony. All the instruments must play together at the same, or appropriate, time, or you won't get the desired results. If you focus solely on the food, or only on the exercise, you're just playing one instrument. The challenge is to get all the instruments playing in unison and you have to keep playing them long enough to create the habit of harmony. The same principles apply in losing weight.

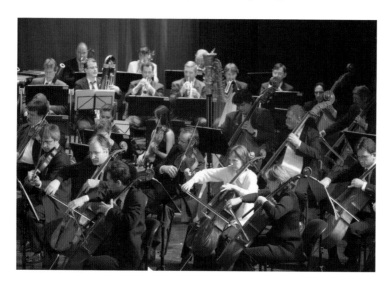

In this book, I will share "my instruments" for lifestyle changes. It's likely that you've heard many of them before, but I will show you strategies for incorporating them into your life. My hope is to motivate you to create and share your own music.

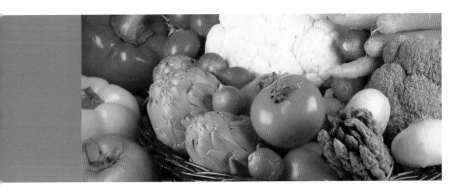

Keys to Optimal Fitness

When you're first starting out, it can be daunting to try to do everything all at once, so don't. Take one step at a time: master one or two keys, and then add one or two more. Here are some key starting points:

1. I eat 1,600 to 1,800 calories a day, broken down into three meals and three snacks. Check with your health specialist first for your optimal calorie intake for weight loss. For a regular fuel injection, eat a meal or a snack every two to three hours.

2. Eat eight servings of fruits and vegetables daily. A serving of fruits or vegetables varies from a half cup to one cup.

3. Limit bread to two servings per day, and choose complex carbohydrates from whole grains, as opposed to refined foods such as sugar and white flour.

4. Consume two tablespoons of healthy oil, such as olive oil or oils found in nuts or vegetables each day. Most oils I use come from meats, fish, salad dressings, and nuts.

5. Exercise thirty minutes to one hour a day six days a week. I always take off one day to rest. Start gradually and work up. Be sure to consult your doctor before starting any exercise program. My program includes three strength-training workouts per week and water aerobics or swimming twice a week. I wear a pedometer and strive to take 10,000 steps a day. I bike ride for fun when the weather is good. If I bike, I decrease my walking. Remember, I have worked up to this regimen over several years.

6. Control stress through planning and the ability to say, "No, I will not be able to do that right now." Say no to requests you do not have time for so you can say yes to your health, weight, and happiness.

7. Get a full night's rest, about seven to eight hours of sleep. I usually go to bed early enough that I can wake up without an alarm.

8. Drink eight cups of water (8 ounces each) daily.

9. Plan and prep your meals. When meats and vegetables are pre-prepped, it's faster and easier to cook a healthy meal. Have every family member share duties during meal preparations.

10. Control portions. Premeasure food items into proper portions so you'll be less tempted to overeat. By weighing and packaging foods ahead of time, you can better control your serving size. When I fail to do this step, I usually get tripped up and end up eating too much.

11. Make yourself accountable. Identify your goals in weekly time periods and write down the steps it will take to accomplish them. Three-month goals let you set your sights a little bit further out. Find someone you trust to check in with once a week to hold you accountable. Keep a daily food and exercise diary. This will help you know whether you are following your program. Without writing these things down, it is easy to lose track, often resulting in weight gain.

12. Enjoy the journey and never, ever give up.

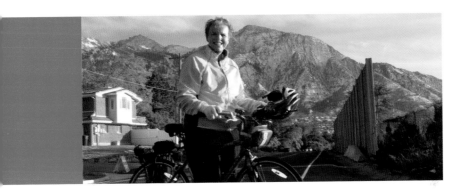

My Journey:
Famous to Fat to Fit and Feeling Fabulous

All of us would love to be able to wave a magic wand over our body, and *voila*! All our excess weight would disappear. For years, Americans have reached for that magic pill, workout device, food or diet, and even "magic" surgery. Yes, all these can bring some results, but in the long run, most of them fail and people end up unhappy and often heavier than before.

Every overweight person must eventually hit that reality point, that final straw, where they say, "This is it. I can't live like this any longer! I'm willing to do whatever it takes to lose the weight and regain my health." You must be willing to make a commitment and stick with it long enough to see results. Then stick with it some more. If you keep flirting with every faddish diet and hoping for short-term magic bullets, you'll never see long-term results.

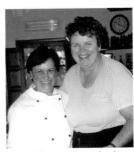

In an Italian cooking school

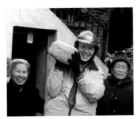

In China

Let me share with you my story of how I got to that 326½-pound tipping point where I was able to make a commitment, and then see what happened.

My Journey

Growing up, I was an adventurous, active, creative child. I was blessed with the good fortune of being raised in the Manti-La Sal National Forest in southeastern Utah, where my father, Julian Thomas, was a district forest ranger.

Life at the ranger station, where my four brothers and I had 240 acres to run, play, and build on, was never dull. I rode my green bike to elementary school in the small town of Monticello. It was a two-mile round trip, and I often rode home for lunch as well. Non-structured exercise, and a lot of it, was just part of our daily life.

Camping and outdoor cooking skills became second nature to me. Our family didn't have a television until we moved to Salt Lake City when I was twelve. As a youth, I was trim and physically fit. But academically I struggled, especially with reading. With the help and encouragement of my parents and teachers, I completed high school, then persevered and graduated from Brigham Young University with a major in home economics. My first full-time job was teaching consumer science at Orem Junior High School. Also, I directed the Brighton Girls Camp located in the Wasatch Mountains near Salt Lake City during the summers. I incorporated outdoor cooking techniques into my lesson plans. I taught my students various skills such as how to make meat loaf in an onion, roast chicken in an underground pit, and cook scrumptious meals in a Dutch oven. During this time I was also very involved in sports and outdoor activities.

After teaching for three years, I returned to BYU for my master's degree in education, and my thesis centered on how to teach outdoor cooking skills in the

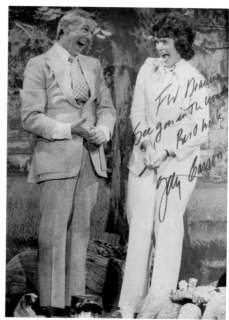

Johnny Carson, 1975

public school system. It was the forerunner of my book *Roughing It Easy.*

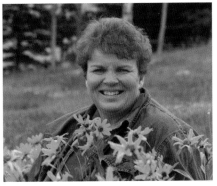

Hiding behind flowers

Roughing It Easy came off the press in March of 1974. I had already been speaking professionally for several years, including tours with BYU Education Week programs throughout the U.S. and Canada. Some years I would travel to thirty cities, interviewing with the media in the mornings and speaking in the afternoons. In 1975, I appeared on *To Tell the Truth, The Mike Douglas Show,* and Johnny Carson's *Tonight* show. At the time, Carson was king of late-night TV. During my sixteen-minute segment on June 5, 1975, I showed him how to start a fire using flashlight batteries and steel wool, and how to "fry" bacon and eggs in a paper sack. Thanks to the national exposure, *Roughing It Easy* went to the top of the New York Times best-seller list.

The book's success and my media exposure propelled me into the heady-but-hectic world of national television, with an eight-year stint as a regular on NBC's *Today* show followed by six years with ABC's *Home Show.* Other highlights of my media career came when I interviewed President Reagan, and I appeared on shows with Regis Philbin, Willard Scott, Martin Short, and Phil Donahue and on ABC's *Good Morning America.*

I was invited to lunches, dinners, and parties. I was frequently invited on food editors' trips that included opportunities to feast on the most incredible delicacies. I didn't want to miss a bite! I ate with reckless abandon.

As a national spokesperson for divisions of Kraft Foods, Procter & Gamble, Dow Chemical, and others, I enjoyed numerous food industry junkets, media dinners, and recipe tastings. Fast food, gourmet food, free food, little exercise, and lots of stress came with this hectic lifestyle. And there was so much work—shows to be planned, books to be written, and presentations to be made. I had always wanted to get married and have a family, but my life instead became consumed by a career that sometimes took me on the road for 300 days a year.

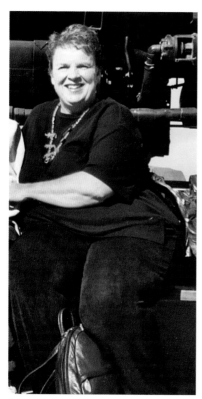
Trip to Mexico, 2003

Food was my occupation as well as my preoccupation and reward system. When I was writing my books I would tell myself, "If you will just read this chapter and correct it, you can go to McDonald's for a Big Mac." My weight crept up along with my stress level. I began one weight-loss program after another. But then I would fall off the wagon, resulting in a cycle that repeated itself for years.

By the mid-1980s, I was experiencing burnout and some depression. One of the side effects of the medication that was prescribed was weight gain. Food was my constant companion, and I used it to keep going with my busy life.

I continued to appear on the *Today* show in New York every other week until 1988. Then I was asked to become a regular member of ABC's *Home Show*. As a talent on the show, I appeared every week for the next six years. The night before the broadcast, I flew from Salt Lake City to Los Angeles, did the show the next morning, and then flew home. I had five days to get the next week's show ready, and then I would start the routine all over again. I loved the show and met the most wonderful people. The audience was about 4 million, roughly the same as the *Today* show, so it was great exposure. The *Home Show* ended in 1995 after six years, and I then became a regular on *Home and Family* on the Family Channel. That lasted for three more years.

In 2000, my aging parents were experiencing health problems and were unable to live on their own. By then my TV career had tapered off, and I moved in with them to become their caregiver, which I did until they died in 2002 and 2004. That was a particularly stressful time for me. I had tried to help my ailing mother gain weight, since she weighed only 95 pounds, but the pounds found me instead.

At a funeral not long after my parents passed away, Floss Waltman, with whom I had worked at Brighton Girls Camp, leaned over to me and whispered, "If you don't lose weight, we will be coming to your funeral soon." That was a bold statement for her to make, but something I needed to hear. If I had continued in the direction I was going, she would probably have been right on the mark.

By now I had been featured in major media for over twenty-five years, and I decided to shift gears and begin a new business. "How to Get a Million Dollars' Worth of Free Publicity" was developed to share the knowledge I had gained in the media spotlight. I created and conducted seminars on how businesses could obtain free media exposure as I had done for twenty-five years.

In the fall of 2003, after speaking at one of these seminars in Santa Monica, California, a participant, Jackie Keller, approached me and said, "I can help you lose weight." She is a wellness coach and founder of NutriFit, a company that delivers customized, nutritious meals.

Her words sparked that hope I had always had of slimming down and enjoying a more active lifestyle. At first I thought she was promoting some multi-level venture and wanted to get me in her program. I thanked her, took her card, and told her I would contact her later. I knew I had a serious problem but, at the time, I just wasn't ready to face it.

My wake-up call came that Christmas. I went to New York City with a friend for the holidays. There was so much to see and do, but my right knee was so weak I could hardly get around in a city designed for walking. We had to take taxicabs almost everywhere. I was sure that a knee replacement was in my near future. I had even considered getting a cane, but my pride wouldn't allow it. I felt like I was falling apart. I was already sleeping on an elevated pillow to alleviate acid reflux at night, I was plagued with a heel spur, and my blood pressure was climbing. I couldn't fit into a regular airplane seat without overflowing into the aisle.

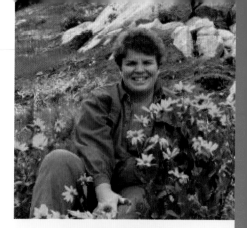

Toward the end of the trip, I was horrified to learn I was now at 320 pounds. I had so much pain and sadness. How could I, a disciplined, hard-working person, have let my body get into this shape? As I flew home I had a lot of quiet time to ponder what I should do. I decided that more than eating all the delicious food I encountered daily, I wanted my health back.

I asked myself:
1. How did I get into this shape?
2. Can I really get myself out?
3. What will it take, and can I get the kind of help I need, since I have not succeeded on my own?

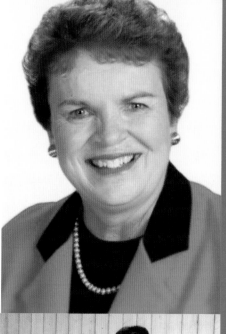

That little spark Jackie Keller kindled was still there. I told myself I didn't have to live a life of pain, inactivity, and desperation.

After landing at the Salt Lake City Airport, I resolved to do whatever it took to lose the extra baggage. I went right home, found Jackie's card, and called her. She agreed to become my wellness coach. That was the beginning of my new life. It had taken me many years to put the weight on, and it took many years to take it off, but it has been a journey worth every step, a journey back to a healthier, happier me.

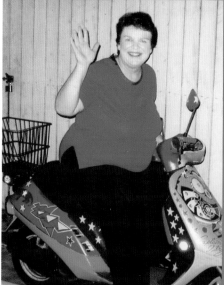

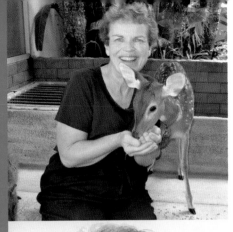

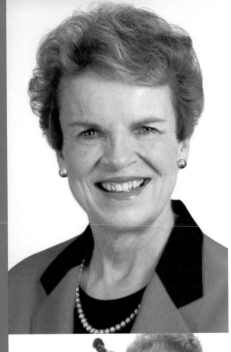

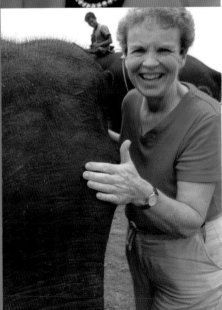

Jackie started me out with the simple basics that most diet regimens require such as planning healthy meals and being more active. My meals contained about 350 to 450 calories each and snacks were 150 calories each. I avoided processed and fried foods in favor of lean meats, complex carbohydrates, fruits, and vegetables.

I assumed I already knew all about nutrition because of my home economics background, but Jackie was a master and added so much excellent new information. For instance, I can still have peanut butter but only one tablespoon of a reduced-calorie kind. Surprisingly, it tastes the same as regular peanut butter to me. I carefully measured it out and just about everything else that I might be tempted to overeat. My refrigerator and cupboards were lined with plastic bags of proportioned foods: four ounces of meat or seafood, half-cups of cooked pasta, snacks of ten almonds plus two tablespoons of dried fruit, and so on.

Because I had portioned and prepped most of my food in advance, I could make myself a meal in under fifteen minutes. That's less time than it took to drive to a fast-food outlet and order at the drive-through. Besides the unneeded calories, I saved time and gas, which were added bonuses.

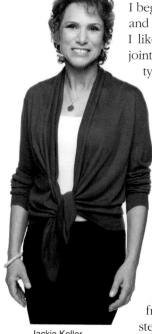

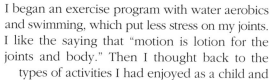

I began an exercise program with water aerobics and swimming, which put less stress on my joints. I like the saying that "motion is lotion for the joints and body." Then I thought back to the types of activities I had enjoyed as a child and remembered my love of bicycle riding. At a local sporting goods store, I happened across a bike sale and splurged and bought two. That way, I reasoned, if a tire went flat on one, I could ride the other while the flat was being repaired. No excuses!

Since then, I've cycled thousands of miles.

Next, I bought a pedometer to gauge the number of steps I took. I researched on-line to find one with the best features for me. My goal was four miles or 10,000 steps per day six days a week. I take one day off from exercise and don't worry about the steps—our bodies need a recovery day.

Jackie Keller

Without question, the biggest challenge was getting all the pieces in place and sticking with them so that I could lose weight consistently. Ten minutes of gluttony, I knew, could do enough damage to set me back several days.

I've been rewarded immensely with good results. After the weight started coming off, I was able to return to the ski slopes for the first time in more than fifteen years. I can walk for blocks without stopping several times to huff and puff. If I'm sitting on the floor, I can stand up without help, and mild exertions that would have been impossible a few years before are no longer a challenge.

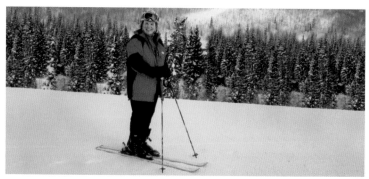

On the slopes

Jackie said she has seen both a mental and physical change in me. "Dian has evolved into a different person. She's definitely come to an understanding of the role of food in her life. She doesn't feel deprived at all. It's such a joy to work with her because you see a new person who transformed herself in more ways than just physically."

For the past four years I've led travel groups to China, first with Morris Murdock Travel, and now with Dick Jensen and Alan McKay Tours. The China tours came about because of my biking. When Dick Jensen was with Morris Murdock, he considered putting together some biking tours. A friend who noticed I was always out biking suggested I would be an ideal tour director. Although the biking tours didn't prove feasible then, I now lead three China tours per year for Dick. Even on my tours I come prepared with prepackaged snacks, and I'm careful about my meals. Now I can fit into my airplane seat just fine.

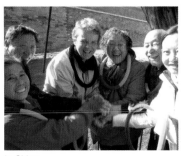
In China

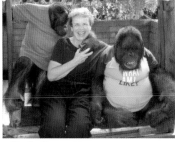
In Thailand

It's not been easy, and I know paying careful attention to my health will be a challenge for the rest of my life. But along the way, I pick up little tips that help me, and when I put them all together, they equal success.

One day last year, I received an e-mail from a woman in California who had heard about my weight loss. She wrote, "You have to write a book. I've got to have help." For months I resisted writing another book because of the challenge it is for me to do it.

My resistance evaporated when Brian Mullahy asked to do a feature story about my weight loss on Salt Lake City's Channel 2 Ten O'Clock News. The next day I got a call from Valerie Phillips, the food editor at the *Deseret News*. She put together a two-page feature story. Then Angie Hutchinson, feature editor from the same paper, asked me to write a column and a weekly blog for the newspaper. At that point I decided if I could write columns and blogs, I could jump back into book writing.

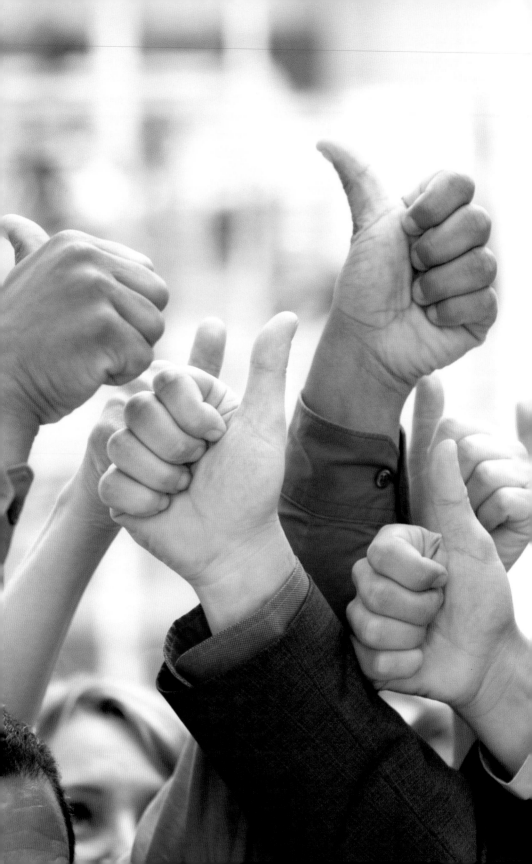

Chapter 2
Emotions

Self-Love Must Come First

Our emotional state is often tied to what we eat and how we feel about ourselves. Self-image and self-confidence are also important parts of the package. As I embarked on book tours with various media, I found myself on a path I never dreamed would be possible for me. On the outside I looked attractive and presentable. I had graduated from BYU, had three successful years of teaching, and was now a successful author and professional speaker.

But underneath, all was not well. My self-esteem suffered because I had always struggled with school. My parents even drove from Salt Lake City to Provo many weekends to read to me as I struggled to complete my university courses. Because I did not do well in school, I sometimes questioned how smart I was.

Success and new-found fame gave me a shot of confidence, and I wanted more and more of it. I wanted people to think I was competent and successful, even though I did not feel it inside. I began to push myself further, piling stress upon stress.

In addition to being a regular on the *Today* show, I was also writing a new book. Television is very competitive, often brutal, and the pressure is intense. If you make one misstep, there are a hundred people waiting to take your place. So I had to be at the top of my game at all times. I was working seventy to eighty hours weekdays, and weekends were rarely my own.

I became depressed and saw a doctor. The medication he prescribed had a side effect of weight gain. I ate more and more to fill the void I felt in my soul.

The frantic pace of my work had to stop, and I was fortunate to find a wonderful therapist. I learned that I was looking outside of myself for the things that I should be giving myself. I must have asked my therapist a thousand times if I was okay.

Once I felt somewhat reprogrammed, I asked her whether she thought I was smart. She would tell me, "I do not know anyone else who has done all that you have accomplished."

Slowly I began to reverse the wrong ideas I had about myself. I learned that I was worthy of respect, and that I was intelligent. I realized I had to love and care enough about myself to do the things required to maximize my health.

With the help of incredible, supportive people, I began to make improvements. I am now very active. I love my new life and the activities that I engage in which were not possible before.

Question: Do you have feelings about yourself that contribute to emotional eating? How can you build your confidence and begin to care more about yourself?

_____

_____

_____

_____

_____

_____

_____

_____

_____

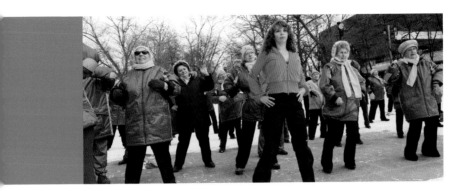

Keeping an Exercise and Food Journal

"Recording everything you eat in a journal is one of the most effective things you can do to lose weight," says Jackie. "Remembering exactly what you put into your mouth makes you more accountable. Keeping a journal also helps you uncover hidden sources of calories and discover emotional eating triggers."

A goal unwritten is only a wish. Here are some examples of goals and plans I've written down, and how I've carried them out.

1. How much do I want to weigh? Write down a realistic target date for reaching that goal. For example, "I want to be 198 pounds by June 1." Weight loss is an individual thing. A plastic surgeon in New York once told me not to lose more than a pound a week, as it takes time for our bodies to change. I averaged a half pound to one pound a week.

2. Make a weekly written plan for three healthy meals and three snacks a day. Once my meals are planned, I shop and prepare foods in advance, so the meals are quick and easy to prepare.

3. A food and exercise journal helps you be accountable to yourself and to your support system. Be honest and share your challenges and successes in it. I weigh myself every day, but Jackie suggests weighing once a week.

Sample entry: *One evening I attended a party where ice cream, sweet rolls, fudge, and chocolate-caramel pretzels were being served. I knew I could not make my goal for that week if I gave in. After I made it through the night successfully, I wrote down the experience in my journal and then e-mailed Jackie. She replied, "Great resolve, keep it up." I also vowed to take my own 150-calorie treat with me to the next gathering.*

4. Visualize accomplishing the goal, and write down three "affirmations" or positive statements that you can vocalize each day. Seeing yourself at the goal line and giving yourself positive feedback will support your outside efforts.

5. I like to plan my weekly exercise and then share it with Jackie. This helps me make the commitment to do the activity.

Success comes through careful planning, being very specific about how you will accomplish your goals, and then writing them down.

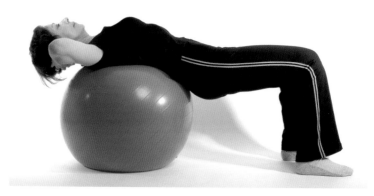

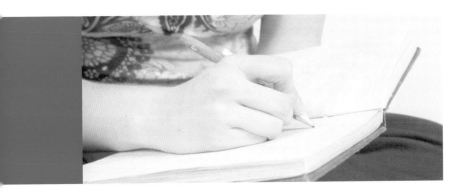

Set Smart Goals

As I was goal-setting early this year, Jackie told me about making SMART goals: Specific, Measurable, Action-Oriented, Realistic, and Timed. She suggested setting three-month goals, rather than a year's worth, and identifying no more than three goals in each of three categories: Nutrition, Exercise, and Lifestyle.

Let me share with you the three-month goals I set for myself and how Jackie responded to them.

Goals from January to April

Nutrition goals:
Dian: Write down everything that I eat.

Jackie: *Not specific enough. Are you using my journal form? I would suggest you also write down when you eat and where you physically are. In other words, are you sitting at the kitchen table, standing in the kitchen, sitting in front of the TV? This information will help you understand your patterns of eating.*

Dian: Nibbling has been a challenge for me. I will write down everything that I eat. I will chew gum to keep myself from piecing when I am preparing food.

Jackie: *Turn this into an affirmative statement: I will chew gum when preparing meals.*

Exercise goals:

Dian: I will keep a daily exercise journal and do three of Rick's (my trainer) routines each week: Tuesday, Thursday, and Saturday.

Jackie: *At what time? If you do the same routine over and over, you won't continue to progress—remember, the workouts need to get progressively more difficult. Three months of the same thing is not progressively more difficult. If you always do what you've always done, you always get what you've always had!*

Dian: Do three water aerobic workouts each week: Monday, Wednesday, and Friday.

Jackie: *Ditto for the above comments.*

Dian: Take 10,000 steps per day, five to six days a week.

Jackie: *Which days will you take off?*

Dian: I will take Sunday off. When the weather is good and I can go biking, then I'll cut the number of steps to 5,000.

Jackie: *How much are you going to ride? Be specific—how long, at what pace, when?*

Lifestyle goals:

Dian: I will plan my days in advance to cut down on stress.

There are still times when I fall off the wagon. No one is perfect 100 percent of the time. When you face challenges, stop and think about what you can do to move forward again. That is just what I do. Then I take Jackie's idea of writing down goals and make them SMART goals:

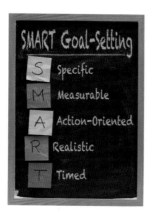

SMART Goal-Setting

S — Specific

M — Measurable

A — Action-Oriented

R — Realistic

T — Timed

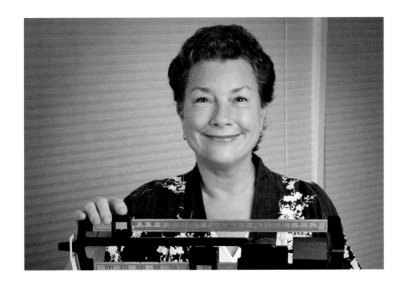

Setting, writing down, and sending my weekly SMART goals to Jackie really helps me to effectively use this five-step process.

Remember that the small steps you take daily make a big difference in your health, your weight, and your happiness.

Question: What are some SMART goals you can make?

_____

_____

_____

_____

_____

_____

_____

_____

_____

_____

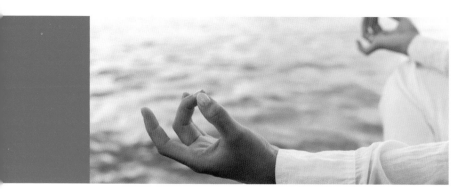

Three P's in a Pod for Stress-Free Living

Challenges are a part of everyday life. It doesn't matter who you are, where you live, or what you do for a living, you will have problems. We can't keep challenges at bay, but we can choose how we deal with them.

Over the years, I've learned to cope with stress and other difficulties by using a formula that I created called "Three P's in a Pod."

1. Keep a POSITIVE mindset.
2. Be open to POSSIBILITIES.
3. Rely on PEOPLE to help and guide you.

1. Keep a POSITIVE mindset

When I was a little girl, every year my parents, my brothers, and I would take a trip to northern Utah to visit my grandparents, aunts, and uncles. We stayed with my aunt who lived near the BYU campus, and Mom and Dad would often take us there. As we walked around the campus, they would smile and say, "This is where you're going to college." "Of course it is," I thought. Unfortunately, not everyone agreed.

In my sophomore year of high school, I took an aptitude test designed to guide my career choice. Shortly after taking the test, I was called in to the school counselor's office. With test scores in hand, Miss Roberts inquired about my post-high school plans. I confidently told her that I was going to attend BYU.

She replied, "I don't think you'll make it. You scored 14 out of a possible 100 in English and 98 out of 100 in problem-solving. You simply don't have the aptitude in English and writing to survive college." She then added that because my problem-solving skills were so high, I might want to consider becoming an auto mechanic.

I decided I was not going to allow another person to dictate the direction of my life. Once I had graduated from high school, I was accepted at BYU. College required a lot of hard work, and it took me five years, not the usual four, to graduate, but I did graduate! Later, I even received my master's degree.

As Henry Ford said, "If you believe you can do something, you can; if you believe you can't, you're probably right."

2. Be open to POSSIBILITIES

This country is known for its many possibilities. In fact, America is often referred to as the land of opportunity—or possibilities. The Pilgrims came for religious freedom, and today many come in search of new possibilities.

Brian Tracy, a self-help author on leadership and business topics, said, "The potential of the average person is like a huge ocean unsailed, a new continent unexplored, a world of possibilities waiting to be released and channeled toward some great good."

In 1944, Frederick Smith was born into a wealthy family. But as the Smith family could tell you, money isn't everything. Fred's father died when Fred was only four years old. He attended Yale University where he wrote a paper for his economics class suggesting the concept of overnight package delivery. The professor wasn't impressed and Fred's grade suffered. After graduation, Fred joined the U.S. Marine Corps, was assigned to fly in Vietnam, and completed two hundred missions.

Fred returned to the States in 1970, still believing in his idea of overnight package delivery. In the early 1970s, he launched Federal Express, which some referred to as "one of the boldest gambles the business world has ever seen." Packages would be flown to Memphis, Tennessee, each night, sorted and flown back out, and then driven to their final destination. The first delivery was in 1973, and today FedEx is a multi-billion-dollar company serving the global transportation business in 220 countries.

William Arthur Ward asserts, "Nothing limits achievement like small thinking; nothing expands possibilities like unleashed imagination."

Always be open to possibilities.

3. Rely on PEOPLE to help and guide you

People can often be the great gateway to success if they are positive, open, and interested. Just as Google built a network of Internet resources, you can build a people network by always taking an interest in others, learning about their skills and talents, and supporting and encouraging them in their goals and aspirations.

Many times the people we meet as we go through life can be bridges to our goals. Daryl Hoole, a longtime friend, introduced me to a man who was assisting her with her Web site, Bill Mansell. As we talked, I learned about Bill's online store. MindPerk is a company that he and his wife, Marquette, created which sells self-help audiobooks all over the world. I discovered that his goals were to be a professional speaker and to write books. We formed an alliance: Bill would help me with my Web site, and I would help him with his first book. As we brainstormed together, it was Marquette who gave me the title for this book. Bill and I have traded services, and now both of us have new books from the support we have given each other.

Sometimes we face problems that we can't solve on our own, one of mine being weight management. Over the years I tried many different weight-loss programs, but I failed at each one. It wasn't until I called Jackie that I was able to rethink being thinner. I can't tell you how glad I am that I didn't block Jackie from my "Google people search."

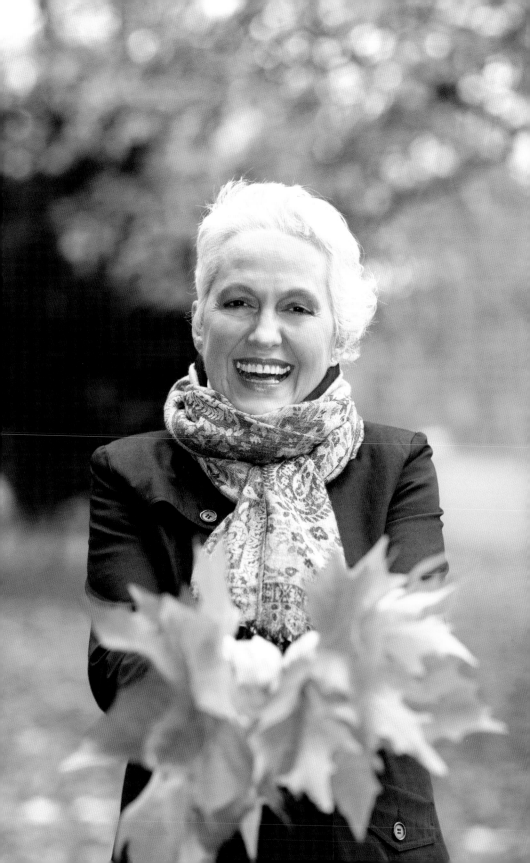

At times there will be things you will feel are impossible to accomplish. Return to your people network and find that "someone" who can support you in your process. When you reach out and let others help you, or you reach out and help someone else, you are both blessed.

An old Chinese proverb says, "When the student is ready, the teacher will appear." It also works in reverse. When the teacher is ready, the student will appear. You will be able to bless many people's lives by reaching out and encouraging them. This will pump air under their wings, and they will fly to places they never dreamed possible. You will also be blessed with a great feeling of satisfaction.

Every morning choose to make it a good day with the "Three P's in a Pod":
1. Keep a POSITIVE mindset.
2. Be open to POSSIBILITIES.
3. Rely on PEOPLE to help and guide you.

Question: What can you do to keep a POSITIVE mindset?

_____

_____

_____

_____

_____

Question: What are the POSSIBILITIES that you have not yet seen?

_____

_____

_____

_____

_____

Question: Who are PEOPLE in your network who can help you, and you can help as well?

_____

_____

_____

_____

_____

_____

_____

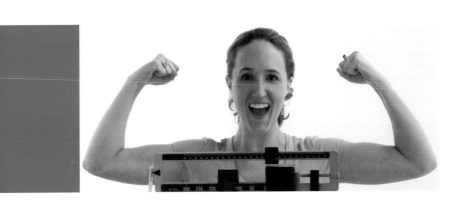

Positive Thinking

Going through the process of losing weight, I found myself reflecting upon my progress at year's end. I knew my weight was up a little from the previous year's and that my weigh-in would come the day after New Year's Eve—not a good night for refraining from food! On Saturday, I woke up about two a.m. worrying about the weigh-in. After all my hard work, to be up a few pounds was not where I wanted to be. I even shed some tears.

Then came the thought, "Why don't you look at what you did right instead of focusing on the few pounds that you've gained?" I was pleasantly surprised. I had been traveling nearly one hundred days of the previous year. Two of my six trips were to Thailand where almost every dish included coconut milk. Those were the trips where my weight slipped up a bit.

I then considered the amount of exercise I had done throughout the past year. In April, May, and June I rode my bike seven hundred miles preparing for my ride across Iowa. Then, at the end of July, I rode 480 miles in one week across the state, and no, Iowa is not flat. One day I even rode one hundred miles! I also passed up numerous pie and ice cream shops along the bike route.

As the New Year began, I felt more encouraged and decided to get up and make a list of the top ten healthy things I had accomplished, which I sent to Jackie. I soon received a note saying, "Great summary!"

Wow! I realized I had focused so much on what the scales read that I forgot to give myself credit for working on my overall health all year. And the proof came when I went for all my medical checkups. It turned out that even though I am a little challenged with my right knee, overall I am still very healthy.

Question: What are the ways that you have improved your health?

_____

_____

_____

_____

_____

_____

_____

_____

_____

Keep Your Eye on Your Goal

We have all watched Oprah slide up and down the weight scale. She can afford to hire anyone to help her, but I believe the most difficult problem she must face is the stress that comes with her demanding schedule. In a similar fashion, my stress increased as I authored books and gained more media exposure. I turned to food for a reward and for comfort.

There are still activities that are very challenging for me. One is traveling. It is hard for me to dine out with friends. When bread is served as an appetizer, it is difficult to stop with one slice. I had to learn to pass up the ice cream and pizza shops in New York. At home, following one weekend trip, I found I had gained a few pounds. When I called Jackie, I told her I thought that I had done pretty well, considering the many opportunities I had for overindulging. What she told me has had a profound effect on me. I have thought of her reply many times.

"If your goal is to lose weight, and if you stayed the same or just went up a little, you did not do very well."

Talk about stopping me in my tracks. Her comment made me redouble my efforts and helped me recommit to my goals.

Question: Are there ways in which you use food as a reward and for comfort? What are things you tell yourself that keep you from reaching your ideal weight?

_____

_____

_____

_____

_____

_____

_____

_____

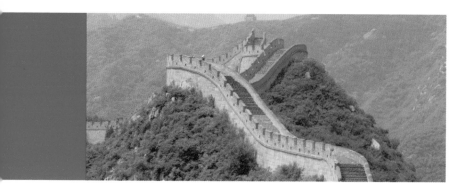

No Limits

How many times are we held back in life because we think we can't do something?

For the past four years, I have led tours to China, and in a recent group one of the participants was a blind man, Premo Foiannini, who, for years, had walked all over Salt Lake City selling brooms.

At the orientation to meet the new travelers, I became very concerned. This was the largest group I had ever led, with forty-six participants. Would I be able to care for them all, including Premo and his wife, Marcelle, who were both in their eighties?

Premo and Marcelle arrived in China the day before we were to climb China's Great Wall. I always stay at the bottom of the Great Wall with those who can't climb steep steps. My right knee lacks cartilage, and I don't climb stairs very well.

I was all set to sit with them and enjoy a few hours of rest and relaxation at the base while the others climbed.

"Would you like to come over here and sit down for a few hours?" I asked.

Premo replied, "Oh, no, we want to walk the Great Wall!"

Astonished at his reply, I shook in amazement and panic. They couldn't possibly go up alone; they could easily take a bad fall. I wanted to make sure they would be safe, so I followed them as they began to ascend the irregular steps. Before I knew it, they were well on their way up.

So, we were off and climbing the steep stairs, Premo and Marcelle and my one bad knee. Every once in a while, as we would stop to rest, I asked Premo, "How far do you want to go?"

"I want to go to the top. You know, there was a blind man who climbed Mount Everest."

I swallowed hard and we continued.

As we neared the third tower, which is well over two-thirds up this particular section of the Wall, you would have thought I was accompanying two rock stars. Tourists from everywhere noticed Premo's white cane and gave him encouraging words and accolades and took his photo as he climbed.

In all of my ten visits to the Wall, this was the highest I had been. I must say, there were a few tears of joy as the three of us reached the third tower.

That day I learned from a sightless eighty-two-year-old near the top of the Great Wall of China that there are no limits to what we can do and where we can go if the desire is there.

Question: What is something you have accomplished, even when others thought it was too hard or impossible?

_____

_____

_____

_____

_____

_____

Question: What is something you would like to accomplish in spite of fears that it's too hard or impossible?

_____

_____

_____

_____

_____

_____

_____

A Winning Game Plan

Recently I was agonizing over the few pounds I had acquired during three weeks in China and Mongolia. A friend said, "Don't worry about the few pounds you put on as long as you keep doing the things you did to lose the weight. You will find that the weight will come off."

This thought relieved the panic and fear that I might be on my way up the scales again. I now know what it takes to lose weight and that the key is conscious effort every day.

I also recalled a time in Florida when I didn't gain an ounce. I weighed in and exercised every day. I ate proper portions of appropriate foods, and I e-mailed Jackie daily for support.

In planning for my most recent trip to China, I worked out the itinerary and made plans to walk more than 12,000 steps each day and to control my food intake. I found a lightweight scale to take with me to occasionally check my progress. Good planning and commitment are always important and necessary and keep me on track.

Know that the weight-loss game is a game you can win. Just like football, there are strategies for winning. Make your winning game plan and stick with it.

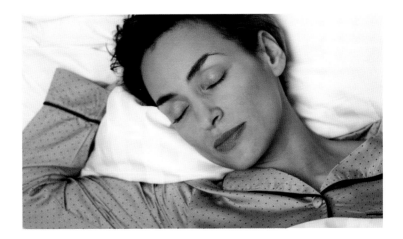

Can Lack of Sleep Affect Your Weight Loss?

As I considered this question, I recalled the many years that I had been writing and making television appearances. I remember the long days that I would put in to get everything done, which resulted in short nights. Often when I became exhausted, I turned to my favorite comfort foods—chips, ice cream, and cookies—all empty, worthless calories.

Several studies have concluded that the less you sleep, the more weight you may gain. A Stanford University School of Medicine study published in 2004 indicates that sleep loss leads to higher levels of a hormone that triggers appetite, and lower levels of a hormone that tells your body it's full. These two hormones—ghrelin and leptin—are thought to play a role in the interaction between short sleep duration and high body mass index. Ghrelin is primarily produced by the stomach and triggers appetite: the more ghrelin you have, the more you want to eat. Leptin, a hormone produced by fat cells, helps control satiety and feelings of fullness.

The bottom line is when you do not get the sleep you need, you often end up eating more—and the wrong kinds of foods.

Since slimming down I have to make sure that I don't get too busy or too stressed, as both drive me to the refrigerator. Good planning is vital to managing my life.

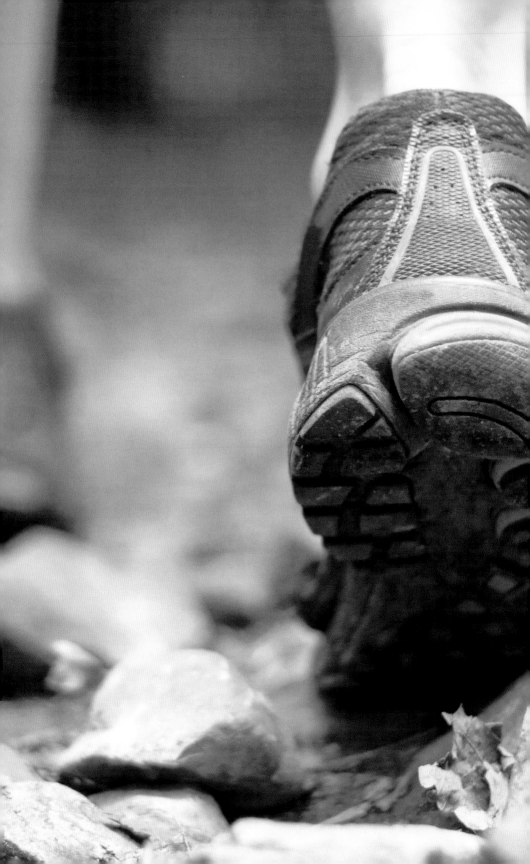

Chapter 3
Exercise

Get Moving!

There are only two times that you have to exercise to lose weight: when you want to, and when you don't. A California friend who gets up and jogs at four a.m. tells me, "I don't like to do it, but I like what it does for me."

Some benefits to exercise:
- It burns calories!
- It helps increase your metabolism so you burn calories at a higher rate, both when working out and at rest.
- It helps release endorphins, which stimulate the pleasure centers in the brain. Hence, you feel better.
- It helps decrease depression. A 2005 study found that walking fast for about thirty-five minutes a day, five times a week, had a significant influence on mild to moderate depression symptoms.
- It helps to keep your blood vessels open and unclogged, decreasing your risk of high blood pressure, elevated cholesterol, diabetes, memory problems, and heart attacks.

One of my weight-loss goals is to work out for at least one hour per day, five days a week. If you aren't exercising at all, start with just ten minutes a day and gradually increase time and intensity. If you overdo it the first few times, you'll end up tired, sore, and discouraged. Be sure to warm up, cool down, and do some stretching to prevent injuries to your joints. You should also consult your doctor before embarking on a vigorous exercise program.

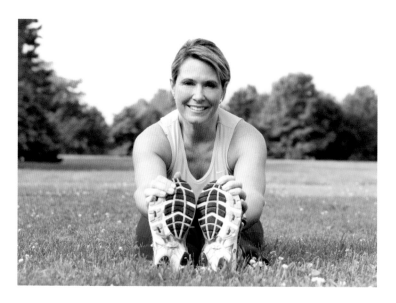

I started with water aerobics and swimming, which were easy on my joints. Later I added biking and other activities.

The Calorie Control Council has a "Get Moving" calculator on its Web site, http://www.caloriecontrol.org/, where you can enter in any type of exercise, the amount of time you plan to do it, and your weight. It will then calculate how many calories you'll burn.

Here is the approximate calorie burn for a 200-pound person doing one hour of the following activities. The calculator doesn't adjust for gender, but men tend to burn calories faster than women, due to their larger muscle mass. Of course, you may not be able to sustain some of these exercises for a full hour, and the calories burned will vary with your weight, how vigorously you exercise, and how many breaks you take.

Aerobics—545
Badminton (singles)—409
Ballet—545
Ballroom dancing, slow—273
Baseball—455
Basketball (half-court)—545
Bicycling, 10 mph—364
Bicycling, 15 mph or vigorous effort—909

Canoeing or kayaking on flat water—455
Dancing, disco—552
Dancing, swing—500
Dusting—227
Frisbee throwing—273
Gardening—431
Golfing without a cart, carrying clubs—500
Grocery shopping—318
Handball—1,091
Hiking—545
Horseback riding—227
Housecleaning—227
Ice hockey—727
Ice skating—636
Ironing—209
Jogging—636
Karate—909
Kickboxing—909
Lacrosse—727
Laundry (folding clothes)—182
Mopping/scrubbing the floor—408
Mowing the lawn—409
Ping-Pong—364
Playing piano—227
Racquetball—636
Raking leaves—364
Rock climbing (ascending)—1,000
Rollerblading—636
Rope jumping—727
Rowing—636
Shoveling snow—545
Snow skiing (cross-country)—727
Snow skiing (downhill)—545
Soccer—636
Spinning (bicycle)—636
Stair climbing—545
Surfing—273
Swimming—545
Tae Kwon Do—909
Tai Chi—364
Tennis (singles)—727
Tennis (doubles)—545
Touch football—732

Vacuuming—227
Volleyball (casual game)—273
Walking briskly—364
Walking the dog or pushing a stroller—227
Washing windows—409
Water aerobics—364
Weight lifting—273
Yoga—364

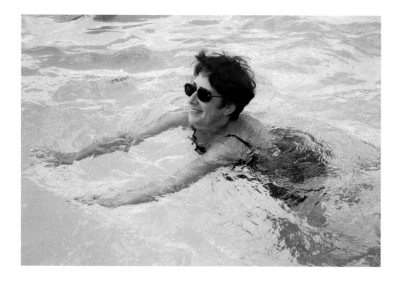

Water Workouts

No matter where you are on the physical fitness spectrum, water is a great place to be.

When I weighed 300-plus pounds, I was too heavy to do much of anything on dry land, but in the water I was buoyant and it supported my joints. This was the perfect place to begin.

Amber Morgan, director of the pool at the Holladay-Lions Fitness and Recreation Center where I work out, said that if you are in waist-high water, it will hold 60 percent of your body weight. When you are chest high, it is 70 percent, and when you are in up to your neck, it holds 80 percent.

Water activities allowed me to ease into exercising. It's a great place to start.

Amber also taught me the five levels of water exercise. If you are a beginner, check with your doctor before starting the first level, and then work your way up. If you are physically strong, start at the level that best fits your ability.

If you're not a swimmer, don't worry. You can stay in the shallow end, wear a foam belt, or use a foam noodle. I have met many people who don't swim but still get a great workout at the pool. Here are the levels you can work through to lose weight and gain greater strength and mobility:

1. Deep water: This is a very low-impact exercise. Some of the movements you can imitate in the water are jogging, bicycling, and cross-country skiing. To stay upright in the water, use a foam belt, life jacket, or foam noodle.

2. Low resistance in shallow water: In this level, you stand waist high and water walk and exercise at the side of the pool. For example, if you want to do push-ups, stand at the edge of the pool, lean out at an angle, then push up; the greater the angle, the greater the resistance.

3. Resistance water: Many pools have a current channel or lazy river, an area where water is jet-forced into a current. You begin by walking with the current and then against it. Being the only one in the current can be extra challenging.

4. Water aerobics classes: Almost every pool offers these exercise classes. I like them because I can move my body in the water in ways that I cannot move on land.

5. Swimming: When you swim at a good pace, you can burn more calories than by running. I have heard experts say that swimming is the best type of exercise there is.

Many people who consider themselves on the plus side hesitate to get into the pool because they are embarrassed to expose their bodies. I decided to do it anyway, because once in the pool, all people can see is your head and a little upper body.

Wear something in which you feel comfortable and not overexposed. Some women prefer shorts and a T-shirt to cover their bulges, or they buy a plus-size swimsuit that provides modest coverage and support so they don't feel as conspicuous. Both www.womanwithin.com and www.roamans.com sell swimsuits and swim dresses up to size 34.

Get started—you'll find that the pool is cool!

Me and My Bike: Find Something You Love Doing

When I got serious about a weight-loss program, I knew I would have to find an exercise that I enjoyed if I was going to stay with it for the long haul. Biking became that exercise.

As a child, I always had a bicycle, almost before I could even depress the pedals. First came a tricycle, and how I loved riding it up and down our driveway! At three, anything that moves you around is thrilling.

In Monticello, Utah, where I grew up, kids usually had the fun of participating in a parade once a year. Our town held parades that commemorated Independence Day and Pioneer Day on July 24th. I was the flag girl and rode my bike proudly out in front, leading the parade as though it were a serious, solemn responsibility.

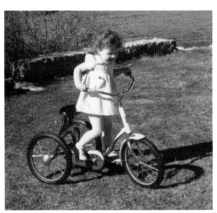

My beginning love affair with bikes.

When I reached the first grade, I wanted a "big kids" bike. My parents knew how much I liked to ride my tricycle, so they ordered me a green one. It did not come with the training wheels, which were ordered separately. I was so excited to have a bike that every night I would persuade my father to hold me steady while I rode it around the house. By the time the training wheels arrived, I didn't need them.

Soon, I was riding my bike everywhere, including to school and my friends' houses which were in town, a far piece from my home at the ranger station. By day's end, I'd ridden several miles; it never once occurred to me that it was beneficial. That's the kind of exercise I love—the kind you do without thinking it's exercise.

After we moved to Salt Lake City when I was twelve, I didn't ride my bike as much, because we lived in a busy neighborhood. When I went away to college, I didn't take my bike with me. My biking days were over—until I needed an activity I could do and enjoy that would support weight loss.

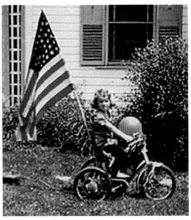
When this trike was decked out with a flag, I was queen of the world.

At that point, I remembered my biking years, and I headed off to a sporting goods store for a recumbent bike. I noticed six of the bikes in the showroom looked just like the one I had as a child. These $300 bikes were on sale for $100 each. I stepped up to the counter and before I knew it I said, "I'll take two."

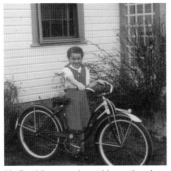
My first bike was almost bigger than I was.

Some time later, I moved up to a fancier lightweight bike that cost many times more than the bikes I bought on sale. Now I ride almost every day, weather permitting. I joined a group of friends who also enjoy cycling. Riding with them has made it so much easier to stay active. As the miles went up, the weight came down.

Many women who have talked to me about exercise say they cannot keep their balance on a bike. I tell them that if the time ever came that I couldn't ride my two-wheeler, I'd just buy an adult three-wheel bike. I want to ride until my last day. I love getting out in the sun and up close and personal with the beautiful country I live in.

Question: What are some of the activities you love doing?

_____

_____

_____

_____

_____

_____

_____

Question: How can you incorporate them into your day?

_____

_____

_____

_____

_____

_____

_____

Step Up Your Exercise Routine

Once it was time to "step up" my exercise routine, I added more steps to my schedule and bought a pedometer. At Amazon.com I read reviews to find the best one to help me achieve my walking goals. I selected the Omron® HJ-112N, which cost less than $30. I keep it in my pocket and use a small fastener to attach it to my slacks, and off I go.

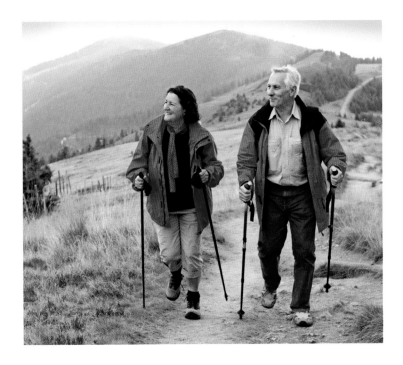

A pedometer senses your body movement and then counts your steps after you have set the length of your stride. It's been a great motivator for me. In fact, one time I became unraveled when the battery died so I bought a backup pedometer, like I did with my bikes. I have walked more in the past year than at any other time in my life.

Research and personal experience have shown me that physical exercise is a major health factor, and walking is one of the best ways to exercise. My pedometer handbook tells me, "For long-term health and reduced chronic disease risk, we should do 10,000 steps a day (equal to four miles). For successful weight loss, this should be between 12,000 and 15,000 steps." This is according to David R. Bassett Jr., a professor in the Department of Health and Exercise Science at the University of Tennessee in Knoxville.

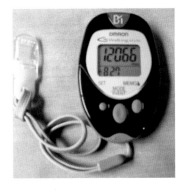

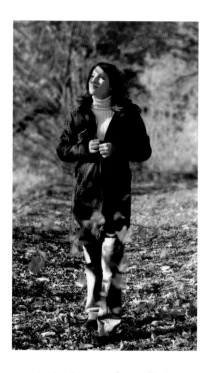

Here are a few additional guidelines from the Surgeon General:

- You don't need special skills or training to be physically active. Start walking; it is a great way to be active.

- Physical activity should be initiated slowly, and the intensity should be increased gradually (e.g., start with a 10-minute walk three times a week and work your way up to thirty minutes of brisk walking or other forms of moderate activity five times a week).

- Activities can be split into several short periods (e.g., ten minutes three times a day) instead of one longer period (e.g., thirty minutes once a day).

- You should select activities that you enjoy and can fit into your daily schedule.

- It may take time to incorporate more activity into your life. Don't get discouraged if at first you miss a day or two; just keep trying to make it a regular part of your routine. You will gradually realize how good it feels to be physically active and fit.

- Ask for support from friends and family; likewise, support the people in your life who are trying to be physically active.

- Many forms of physical activity can be social, allowing you to converse and spend time with family or friends or to develop new relationships.

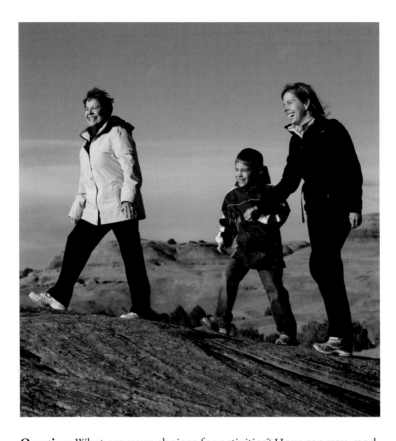

Question: What are your choices for activities? How can you modify your schedule to accommodate exercise?

_____

_____

_____

_____

_____

_____

_____

_____

_____

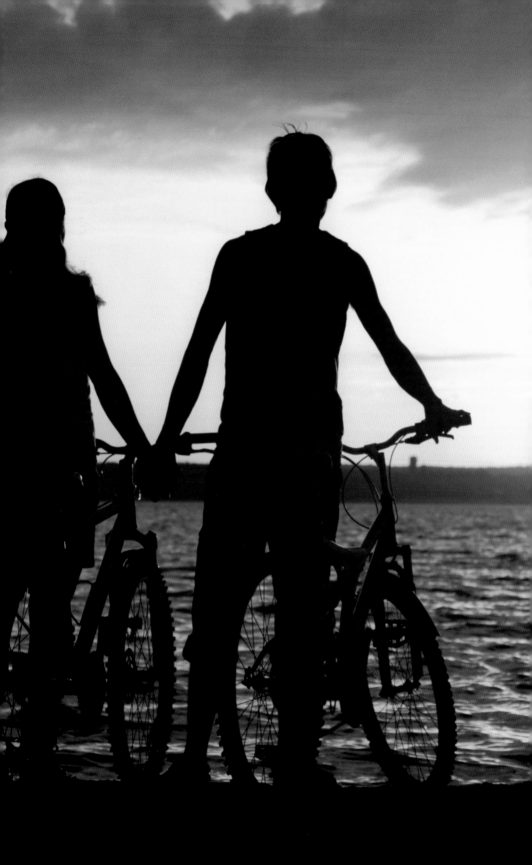

Strength Training

Surveys have identified that the top New Year's resolution every year is to lose weight. In January, the exercise facilities are packed, but by February attendance is back to normal because most people lack commitment and fail to develop a routine that keeps exercise in their lifestyle. The goal of any exercise program is to develop a routine that you can follow.

Strength training—also known as weight lifting or resistance exercise—makes your muscles stronger. When you are pulling or pushing some type of weight, you create tiny tears in your muscle fibers. Your body reacts by repairing those tiny tears and making them bigger and stronger, creating more muscle mass.

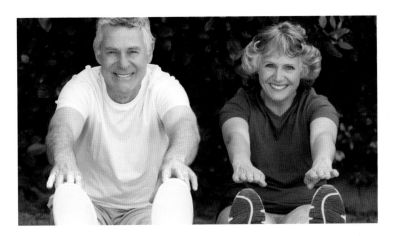

Dr. Phil Allsen, professor of exercise science at Brigham Young University, said, "One pound of muscle at rest requires three times the amount of energy as one pound of fat. During rest, over 70 percent of the energy required by the body comes from stored fat. By increasing your muscle tissue with strength-training programs, you now have a method to increase the uses of stored fat twenty-four hours a day."

Rick Barke, my trainer, said, "Maintaining your fitness varies depending on what type of activity you are engaging in. It also depends on the fitness level you are trying to maintain. Generally speaking, you should be performing similar activities in intensity to the ones you have done to become fit. To become more fit you need to increase your repetitions or the weight. It is always good to consult a professional."

Strength training is key to helping us carry out our daily activities such as lifting groceries, climbing stairs, or pushing a lawn mower. It also helps prevent osteoporosis or brittle bones because it stimulates bone cells to produce more bone.

You're never too old to benefit from strength training. A Tufts University study found that even nursing home residents improved their muscle strength, walking speed, and ability to climb stairs after ten weeks of a strength-training program.

Strength-training can involve dumbbells, machines, elastic bands, or your own body weight. Efficient strength training comes from working the big muscles of your legs, upper body, and abdominals. Balance training with the small muscle groups is also critical, especially if you get more aggressive about using heavier weights. A general rule of thumb is to allow a day in between strength-training sessions to give your muscles recovery time.

When you're just getting started, consider your age, health, and current strength level. If you belong to a gym, ask a trainer to show you around the weight room to identify each machine and demonstrate how to use it. You may want to schedule a session with a personal trainer to assess your fitness level and customize a program for you to follow. There are many ways to get strength training. Do not think that you have to go to a gym. I have developed a routine that I can do with elastic bands and a few simple exercise tools when I am on the road.

If you are over sixty, many senior center, community, or college outreach programs provide special activities and exercise routines designed for your age and activity levels. There are also many classes, instructional DVDs, books, and online guides that show specific strength-training exercises to help you get started and keep going.

Muscle fatigue is normal if you're starting a new workout program. But sharp, jarring, grating, popping, or grinding pains signal trouble. Discontinue that particular exercise and consult your physician.

Functional Exercise

Functional exercise is any task that you do that requires you to use your body and your muscles. The more you do, the better the workout.

Functional exercise came into play in my life last year when my renters of several years decided to move. The duplex needed many repairs. In the past, I had always hired a contractor. A friend suggested that I do the work myself. I am somewhat handy, but was I really competent enough for this big project? It had to be done in a month, in time for new tenants. I decided to go for it.

True, I did hire people to help me, but I was on the job eight to ten hours a day working alongside them. I helped tile the bathroom floor and shower, then the kitchen and entry floors. I also painted walls and ceilings and helped on dozens of other tasks. I was the key shopper which required miles of walking in the home improvement stores. It was some of the hardest physical labor I have ever done, but at the end of the month, I was in better shape, had a beautifully remodeled duplex, and had money in my pocket.

Since that day I look for tasks I can do that provide both exercise and an opportunity to save money. Here are a few things I now do for myself.

1. Shoveling snow: I shovel my walks instead of using my snowblower. When we get a lot of snowfall, I shovel several times during the storm. I dress warmly, work up a light sweat, and enjoy the winter landscape and falling snow. My brother stopped by during a recent snowstorm, while I was out shoveling walks. He said, "What's wrong with your snowblower?" I smiled and said, "I am the new snowblower."

2. Organizing and cleaning: Often when I don't want to go to the gym, I give myself a day of functional exercise. In the process of putting things away and reorganizing areas, I have walked as many as 10,000 steps without leaving my house. For years, I hired cleaning help because I just didn't think I had time to accomplish household tasks. Now I am my own house cleaner and only bring help in when I am overtaxed (especially while writing).

3. Doing yard work: One day my neighbor asked me, "Why don't you get someone to mow your lawn?" I said, "I don't want to pay someone $35 to mow my lawn while I go to the gym and walk the same distance." I have found that I walk a mile in the process of mowing.

4. Organizing my closets: I remove everything from my closet and only put back what I need. This job requires a lot of walking—taking things out and putting them back, tossing out the unnecessary, and stowing the rest in their proper places. The days that I do this, I end up taking 5,000 to 10,000 steps.

5. Running daily errands: Some days when I've cleaned house and run errands wearing my pedometer, I've found that I've taken over 10,000 steps by the end of the day. When I shop, I like to park at the furthest section of the parking lot and walk to the store.

6. Remodeling my house: I am remodeling my basement, and that is where my functional exercise will be focused for the next year. A neighbor, who will help me in the evenings, has agreed to teach me as he performs the tasks that I lack the skill or muscle power to do.

7. Gardening: One of the best functional exercises during the summer and fall is gardening. Not only do you bend and lift, but you also have delicious, home-grown vegetables and fruits to eat.

A good way to start your own functional exercise program is to list what needs to be done around your house and yard, prioritize it, and get to working and walking. Painting, cleaning, gardening, and shoveling snow are just a few chores that can give you a great workout. Mix in a few gym, pool, and weight-training exercises, and you can really become fit.

Question: What are some tasks you can do each day that will add exercise benefits?

_____

_____

_____

_____

Make It Fun!

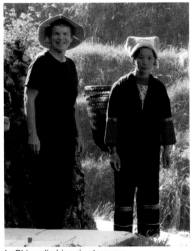

In China climbing rice terraces

As America's choices in entertainment have changed over the years, so have the national obesity rates. Ask your grandparents what they did with their friends for fun. Chances are a night on the town included ballroom or country dancing, or skating at a local pond or rink. If they lived in a rural area, there might have been horseback riding or swimming at a lake.

Growing up at the Baker Ranger Station, we ran around the hills and yard playing, riding our bikes, feeding the chickens, and working in the garden. I recently returned to our old home near Monticello. Some teenagers visiting from the city were in the living room playing video games. I asked them whether they were having fun at the ranger station. They told me they were bored because there was nothing to do. I couldn't believe it! In my day it had been a kids' playground paradise. Many kids today are content pushing buttons for entertainment.

Nowadays when people get together with friends or family, it's often to watch TV or movies, go out to eat, or watch a sporting event. These are all sedentary activities—unless you're jumping up and cheering for your team a lot. Cable TV and DVDs offer endless viewing choices, and the Internet makes it easy to sit at the computer for hours of social networking.

Think back on the disco era of the seventies when everyone was hitting the dance floor á la John Travolta. Now we sit on the sofa and watch *Dancing with the Stars*.

The next time you're planning a family outing, date night, or get-together with friends, consider some active options. You don't need to turn it into a major workout with everyone perspiring, just have enough action to get people moving a little. You won't just be helping yourself, but you'll be helping others to put more movement in their lives.

1. Turn on your Wii or Kinect and do "Just Dance," "Wii Tennis," or one of the many other video "exergames" on the market. Last year, the American Council on Exercise named exergaming one of the top 10 fitness trends. Users find that the more enjoyable the game, the less you notice you are exercising. There are hundreds of activities that cater to all different personalities and activity preferences.

2. Head to a park with a volleyball net or set up one in your backyard.

3. Plant a garden and grow your own vegetables, fruits, and herbs.

4. Mow the lawn.

5. Dust off your tennis racquet and head to a public court.

6. Go bowling or play miniature golf.

7. Try ice or roller-skating.

8. Go for a walk at dusk and watch the sunset, or walk with a friend, your kids, or your grandchildren for some happy one-on-one time.

Question: What are some energizing activities you can suggest for outings with family and friends?

_____

_____

_____

_____

_____

Adding the Social Element

Another key to getting lots of exercise is finding a sport with a social element. There are many activities that you can get involved in with others, such as walking, biking, and dancing. Many cities have clubs for square dancing or country line dancing. Strut your stuff on the dance floor.

Meet a friend and tread water in a pool while enjoying great conversation. There is a group of people who come to my fitness center pool and tread water every day. Besides treading water, they enjoy socializing as well.

I looked for a bicycle group I could participate with. That's when I heard about Ragbrai, the largest bike ride in the world. Two reporters who pedaled across Iowa to collect stories for the newspaper started Ragbrai, the *Des Moines Register*'s Annual Great Bicycle Ride Across Iowa. It has grown to include more than 15,000 riders. It's a cross between the Tour de France, Mardi Gras, and a county fair. As soon as I could, I signed on.

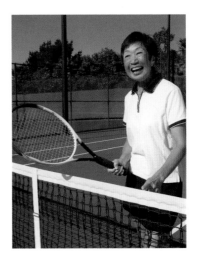

Riders start in western Iowa by backing their rear tire into the Missouri River. They then spend seven days biking across the state to the Mississippi River, where they dip their front tire into the water. The total ride is usually between 440 and 480 miles, depending on the designated route. Each leg varies from a low of fifty miles to a high of eighty-two miles.

At my first Ragbrai, I was fifty pounds heavier and able to ride only 300 miles. The second time, after losing twenty pounds, I rode 330 miles. After I lost another thirty pounds, the third time was a charm. I rode every one of the 480 miles!

Riders come from all across the United States and many foreign countries. One of the greatest benefits of Ragbrai is all the advance preparation for the event. I worked out in the gym, walked many miles, and rode my bike about 700 miles to prepare. With the 15,000 riders and 5,000 support people, the event is a city on wheels. This last year, we started in Sioux City on the west and rode to Dubuque on the east. It is a spectacular adventure, as you can see from the photos.

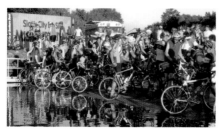
Riders dip their rear tires into the Missouri River.

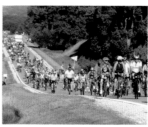
Thousands of bicyclists begin their trek up the first hill of the ride.

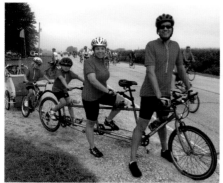
A family of six rode together all the way. The children's ages ranged from one to eight. Two are in the little trailer in the back.

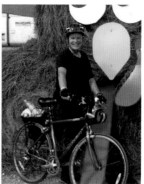
Several towns along the way put up zany decorations for the riders to enjoy.

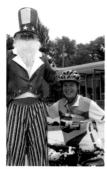
You never know who you'll meet along the way.

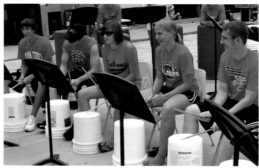
A band entertains riders with bucket drums.

I encourage you to think about what you can turn into a group activity. Many people enjoy being in "fun runs" or even training for marathons or triathlons. Others get in the groove with a yoga, spinning, or aerobics class.

The Huntsman Senior Games in St. George, Utah, offer a variety of sports events each October. Over 10,000 people from all over the world, ages fifty to ninety, gather to enjoy two weeks of over thirty different competitions.

Two years ago, I showed up at the Games and won three gold medals and one bronze. The first bike race was up Snow Canyon. The hill was far too steep for me to ride, so I walked my bike up most of the way. When I made it back down to the bottom, I noticed it had taken most of the riders only twenty minutes to make the ride up while it had taken me over an hour. I suppose stopping along the way to talk to two men had not helped my time. I decided to leave as I knew there was no way I was in the running for a medal. As I started to leave, someone said, "You should check the winners' board before you go. Maybe you won a medal." I just chuckled but decided to follow her advice. As I neared the award area, I heard my name being called out as a gold-medal winner. I was shocked! Later I learned that I was the only participant in that category. What I realized is that sometimes just by showing up you can win a gold medal.

The two men I stopped and talked with became my biggest fans during the week. They arrived at the end of every race to see how I had done. I got so many pats on the back because the "fat lady," me, showed up with all the skinny riders to participate and finish the races. One woman even said, "I sure wish I had the courage to do what you have done. I feel too self-conscious about my weight." I had a ball all week, and it would have been sad to have missed this opportunity because of my weight. I even attended the awards banquet and received a Games T-shirt, which I now wear often, feeling proud and pleased with my accomplishments. It brings back special memories of the week I pushed myself out of my comfort zone.

Question: What types of group activities would you enjoy doing?

_____

_____

_____

_____

_____

_____

_____

_____

_____

No Time to Exercise?

If finding a block of time to devote to exercise is difficult, you can always find small moments to slip in extra steps. For instance, a recent travel day canceled my gym time. What a perfect opportunity to turn my wait time into walk time.

At the airport I had several minutes to walk around the gate area before my flight. After landing, I had to wait for my hotel shuttle so I strolled up and down the sidewalk, keeping an eye on my luggage, until the shuttle came. I actually clocked a mile.

Relaxing in my room that evening, I watched a TV program. Each time a commercial came on, I hopped out of my chair and walked up and down the hall. By the end of the two-hour show, I had clocked another mile. The double benefit was the thrill of missing the commercials!

I shared this experience with a hypnotherapist friend, who told me creative exercise stories about three of his clients.

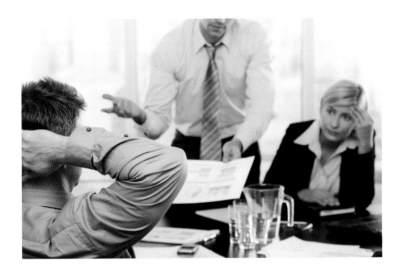

His first client lived on the twenty-third floor of a high-rise. She started exercising after work by taking the elevator to the eighteenth floor and then walking the rest of the way up to her apartment. Each week she would drop down a floor until she was walking all the way up from the fourth floor of the building.

His second client, a woman with small children, lived in a two-story house and decided that each time she had to go up or down the stairs, she would do so six times before beginning her task. Both clients were successful in losing weight by creating maximum exercise in limited time.

His third client took her fifteen-minute work break every day outside in good weather and would walk around the very large building. She also went out for fifteen minutes after lunch. She told him that if she didn't take advantage of those few minutes, she would never get any exercise.

I recently took a five-hour road trip from Salt Lake City to St. George, Utah. There happened to be a town about every sixty miles. In earlier times, the towns were laid out that way, since that is how far an oxen-pulled wagon could travel in a day. I exited at several of the towns and got out to take a five-minute walk to keep myself awake and alert.

A friend recently took his belt down a few notches. I asked him what he did that made the difference. He said, "I simply take the stairs instead of the elevator at work, and I walk every chance I get on the job."

Just start small and work up. Begin with ten to fifteen minutes of activity each day. My thinking has changed since I began losing weight, and I look for ways to be more active.

Think about your day. Is there a break time at work when you could go for a quick walk? Maybe you can slip in ten to fifteen minutes of activity at lunchtime. If you're driving the kids to and from school, perhaps you could walk around the grounds while waiting to pick them up.

Once you decide to become more active, begin looking for additional time for aerobic and weight-lifting exercise such as adding a treadmill or weight bench where you watch TV.

Remember, small steps make huge differences in your health, your weight, and your outlook.

Question: Where can you find opportunities in your day to sneak in a few minutes of exercise?

_____

_____

_____

_____

_____

_____

_____

_____

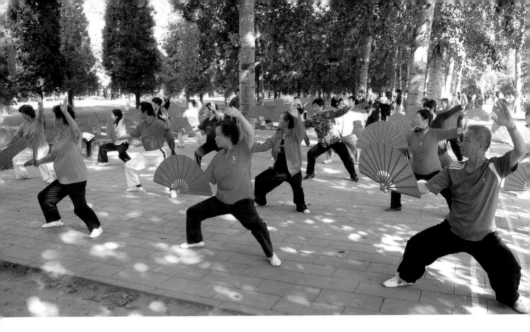

The Chinese Lifestyle

When I travel, I am always looking for the interesting new—and age-old—ways people live their lives.

While leading tour groups to China, I've noticed that it's very rare to see an obese Chinese person. A book I've enjoyed, *The China Study*, explores the benefits of the Chinese lifestyle. Very few Chinese are overweight due to their diet and exercise habits.

It is hard to make a sweeping statement about a population of more than a billion people, but after twelve trips to that country, I can say that the Chinese people, as a whole, have certain in-grained habits that promote health. Here are a few of them we Americans could incorporate:

1. Vegetables are a major part of their diet. Seventy-five percent of any meal in China is usually some combination of many varieties of vegetables, with little added protein. I will often ask, "What is this vegetable called?" "It is a green," will be their reply. I have never seen many of their vegetables before.

I dined several times with a Chinese family who have a seven-year-old boy. He ate every vegetable placed before him, and there were many. You can find a wide variety of fruits and vegetables for every meal, and you never need to leave the table hungry.

2. Meat is a condiment. The Chinese use very little meat. While in

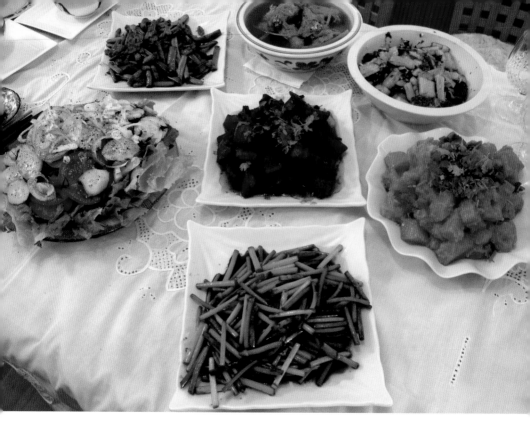

China, I never sit down to a juicy steak. The three protein sources that I see most often are chicken, pork, and fish, which are usually minced and added to a vegetable dish. Occasionally, they may have a skinny free-range chicken with vegetables and broth as a soup. Fish is the exception and is often cooked and served whole.

3. Dessert is fruit. At the end of the meal, you may be served a plate of sliced watermelon or oranges. Most of my Chinese friends don't even like sweet foods.

4. Milk, cheese, and other dairy products are not a part of the Chinese diet. In over a dozen trips there, I cannot recall ever being served dairy products when I eat with my Chinese friends. They are not at all accustomed to dairy in their diet.

5. Breads are rarely served. If you see any type of bread, it will be steamed, as the Chinese kitchen does not have an oven for baking. This steamed bread is like a bun, often containing a filling of sweet pork or bean paste. Woks are the cooking appliance of choice.

6. Fresh is king in China. In the village where I lived for two months, the vegetables I ate were picked that morning and sold at market the same day. Many homes do not have refrigerators, so people must purchase just enough food for that day. There are several farmers' markets in every city. Meats are also purchased fresh daily. In a country restaurant, you choose your favorite live fish or chicken for your meal; after about thirty minutes, it will appear on your plate.

7. Carbohydrates come from rice or noodles. Rice in the south and noodles in the north give the Chinese the energy they need for the day. And they do need a lot of energy, since only about 10 percent have cars. Most ride a bike, walk, or use public transportation.

8. Junk food is not part of the daily intake. None of the Chinese people I know there eat unhealthy snacks. Health is top-of-mind in China; I would say taste and convenience are top-of-mind in America.

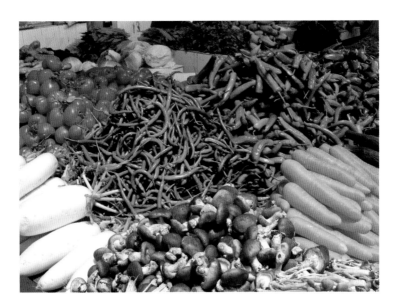

9. Tea and warm water are the drinks of choice. You can find carbonated drinks in China, but I never saw any of my friends drink them—or even drink anything cold. You can't get ice water at a restaurant; instead, you are served hot water or tea.

10. Fast-food consumption is a rare experience. I believe most Chinese people have had a taste of American fast food, but that's about all. They do have Chinese fast food, but it appears to be healthier than American burgers and fries. Unfortunately, with the arrival of Western food and the lure of McDonald's, KFC, and Pizza Hut, more of the young people in China are starting to put on weight.

11. In China, almost all foods are diced or minced before cooking. I was told the reason for this is that in earlier times, firewood was scarce, and the food required less cooking fuel if chopped into small pieces.

12. Exercise is a way of life. The largest and most impressive group of exercisers I've ever seen was in Beijing, China. The Temple of Heaven is a huge park similar to New York City's Central Park. Every day of the year, 50 to 60 thousand people show up to enjoy exercise, fun, and friends. Exercising in the parks throughout the country is an established practice in a senior citizen's daily life. Men and women in China retire at sixty and it is their responsibility to keep themselves healthy. I am always amazed to see how mobile, fit, and flexible they are. I have seen sixty- and seventy-year-olds doing what I have observed only active children in America doing.

A few years ago while visiting China for a month, I guided several tour groups through the Temple of Heaven to watch the Chinese exercise. At that time I weighed about 240 pounds. Each time I would pass through the park, I would see a woman in her sixties who stood about five feet tall. I did not speak Chinese and she did not speak English. But during one of our encounters she placed her hands on the outer sides of my thighs and then moved her hands closer together showing me that I could lose weight. She then walked me over to a fence and showed me how to put my leg up on the rail and move it back and forth. She demonstrated how to pat my legs from top to bottom. It was my guess that both of these activities increased circulation, although I'm not sure because of the language barrier.

I returned the following year, having lost more than thirty-five pounds. When I saw her again, she lit up like a candle and ran over and gave me a huge hug. She was thrilled that I had taken her advice and lost weight.

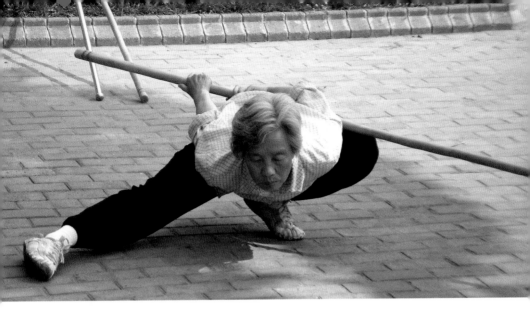

13. They enjoy a variety of activities. One night as our tour group left a restaurant in Xian, we encountered a group of fifty-plus people on a side street line dancing.

As you visit the parks in China, you will observe people performing exercises called Tai Chi sword, Tai Chi ball, and Tai Chi fan. I have also participated with them in several other games that I've not seen anywhere in America. The games are designed to keep participants moving and connecting with each other. When I stop and play with them, I am always amazed at how quickly the time passes.

One day I stopped in a Shanghai park and watched several people play badminton. Seeing me on the sidelines, they motioned for me to come and play with them. I took them up on the offer.

It had been more than thirty years since I had played badminton. As I progressed enough to hit the birdie over the net several times, they beamed and said, "Gooda, gooda." I knew they were happy to play with me and to see me improve. After an hour and a half, I was exhausted. They all gathered around and said to me, "Tomorrow, tomorrow." They wanted me to come back and play again.

14. China is the bike capital of the world. In China I knew I had found my bike soul mates. China has the world's largest bike count. In Beijing there are 16 million people and 10 million bikes. They even have bike lanes with bike stoplights. I was so amazed by what they can load onto a bike. For many, it is their only transportation. Those who aren't bikers are pedestrians.

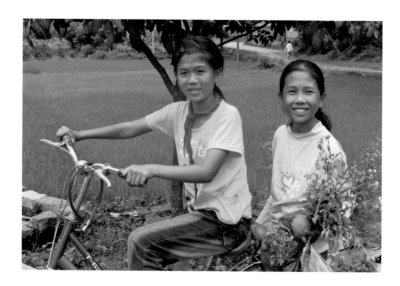

15. The Chinese diet is more varied. It is always a treat to visit their markets and see all the varieties of foods. They also know which foods to eat to make hearts healthier. A restaurant I frequented had a special page just of healthy soups. There were soups for your kidneys, heart, liver, and just about any body system you can name.

In China everyone's health is a major priority. It would be difficult to find a country of that—or any—size that is as concerned about a healthful lifestyle for its people.

Question: What are some of the habits of the Chinese that you can adopt in your own life?

_____

_____

_____

_____

_____

_____

_____

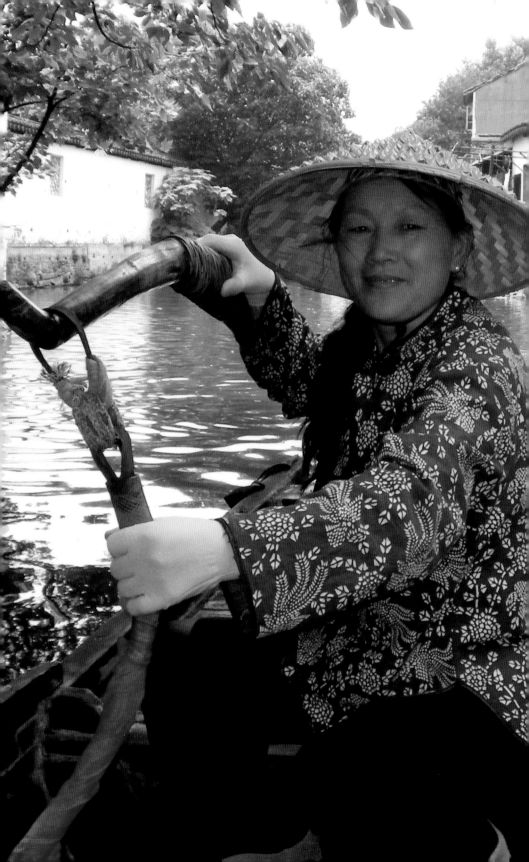

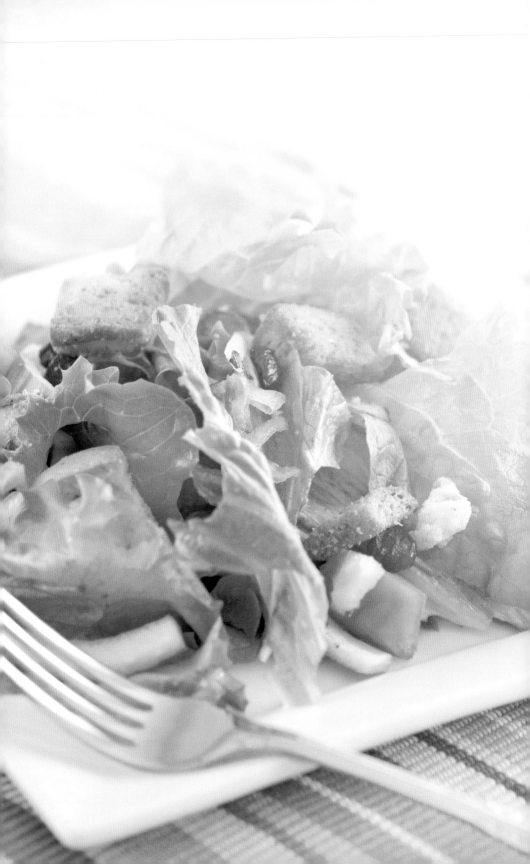

Chapter 4
Nutrition

The Basics

The most important thing that I decided to do for better health was not to diet, but rather to develop a new lifestyle. I learned to eat nutrient-dense foods to keep me from getting hungry and to promote my optimal health. I function well on 1,600 to 1,800 calories per day.

Calorie budgets vary according to weight, body composition, and activity level. One handy way to approximate your daily caloric budget and food intake is to use the USDA's Web site, http://www.mypyramid.gov/mypyramid/index.aspx. There you can enter your age, height, gender, and activity level, and receive an instant calculation of the number of calories you need to maintain an appropriate weight. Remember that each person will burn calories a little differently.

Your overall daily food intake should include:

- **Two servings of protein** (a serving is four ounces raw or three ounces cooked). This includes more than just meats, poultry, and seafood; eggs, dried peas and beans, nuts, seeds, and soy products are also great sources of good-quality protein.

- **Six to eight servings of fruits and vegetables** (a serving is one piece of fruit such as an apple or a banana, one-half cup fruit or vegetables, one-half cup fruit juice, or one cup raw leafy greens). I eat four to six servings of vegetables and three to four servings of fruit each day. I make them the centerpiece of my meals, since they supply the most nutrients for the fewest calories. Starchy vegetables such as potatoes, corn, and peas should be eaten in moderation, no more than a one-half-cup serving per day, but you can have as many servings of nonstarchy vegetables as you like—the more, the better. It is important to eat a wide variety of fruits and vegetables, since each one provides different vitamins, minerals, and antioxidants.

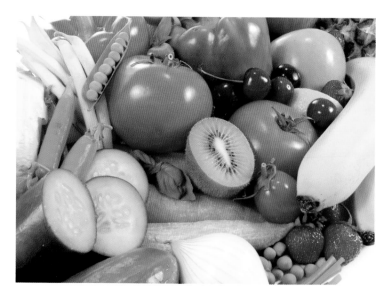

- **Three servings of nonfat or low-fat dairy products** or fortified soy milk (a serving is one cup fat-free milk or yogurt, one-half cup low-fat or fat-free cottage cheese, or one ounce cheese). Avoid yogurt that is sweetened with high-fructose corn syrup or a lot of added sugar. I eat plain, nonfat yogurt and add my own fresh fruit.

- **Six servings of grains** (a serving is one slice of bread, one small muffin, one-half bagel, one-half cup cooked rice or pasta, or one ounce breakfast cereal). Most Americans consume plenty of grains, but not enough whole grains. Processed foods such as white bread, white rice, and pasta have had the bran and many important nutrients removed. Whole grains include the whole package: fiber and naturally occurring vitamins and minerals. I always choose whole-grain products, such as whole-wheat bread or bran cereal. Be sure to watch portion sizes—this is one place that calories can really add up.

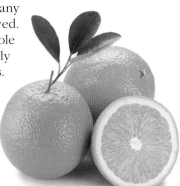

- **Two tablespoons of healthy oils,** as they can be good sources of heart-healthy omega-3 and omega-6 fatty acids. They are also the best substitutes for saturated fats and trans fats, which contribute to heart disease. Olive, canola, or other vegetable oils are good choices. I use Smart Balance Light instead of butter. It is made with healthy oils such as olive oil, flaxseed oil, etc. Oils are high in calories, so use sparingly.

I eat three meals and three snacks daily. This keeps my metabolism fueled all the time, and I'm energized for exercise and activity. My blood sugar stays steady, and I rarely ever get hungry or feel tempted to have one of those "blowout" meals. Eating at regular times establishes a pattern that helps prevent impulse eating.

Give away any junk food you may have in your house. I don't buy foods I shouldn't eat, because if they are in my pantry, I will be sorely tempted. If the people you live with want foods that you choose not to eat, work out a compromise to at least keep them out of sight.

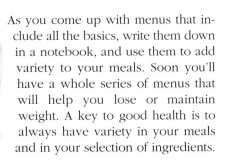

As you come up with menus that include all the basics, write them down in a notebook, and use them to add variety to your meals. Soon you'll have a whole series of menus that will help you lose or maintain weight. A key to good health is to always have variety in your meals and in your selection of ingredients.

Here is a one-day sample menu that invites variety:

Breakfast: 1 to 2 scrambled eggs, 1 slice of whole-wheat toast, ½ cup salsa, and an orange.

Snack: 1 apple with 1 tablespoon reduced-calorie peanut butter.

Lunch: 2 cups homemade chicken vegetable soup and 1 slice of whole-wheat toast.

Snack: 1 cup nonfat yogurt and ½ cup pineapple.

Dinner: 3 ounces cooked pork loin, 1 cup mixed steamed vegetables, ½ cup cooked sweet potato, and 1½ cups spring greens salad with 2 tablespoons Newman's Own Lighten Up Low Fat Sesame Ginger Dressing.

Snack: 1 sliced frozen banana, 1½ cups light vanilla soy milk, and ½ teaspoon vanilla (for banana shake).

Read Labels

The Nutrition Facts label and the ingredients list on packages of foods and beverages are useful tools to help you make choices about the foods you purchase, but don't fall for the hype on the front of the package. Some claims can be misleading. Always check the Nutrition Facts label located on the side or back of the package.

Some of the things you'll learn:

1. The serving size and number of servings in the package: This is important, because the calories, fat grams, etc., are based on the serving size. For instance, a small bag of peanuts might actually contain TWO servings. A pizza that looks like it's enough for only four people might actually contain five or six servings.

2. Calories: This is the number of calories per serving. If the label says a serving is one-half cup and the package contains two servings, you will get twice the number of calories if you eat the whole thing.

3. Calories from fat: If a serving of potato chips is 130 calories, with 80 calories from fat, it may not be a wise choice. Most of the foods you choose should get no more than one-third of their calories from fat.

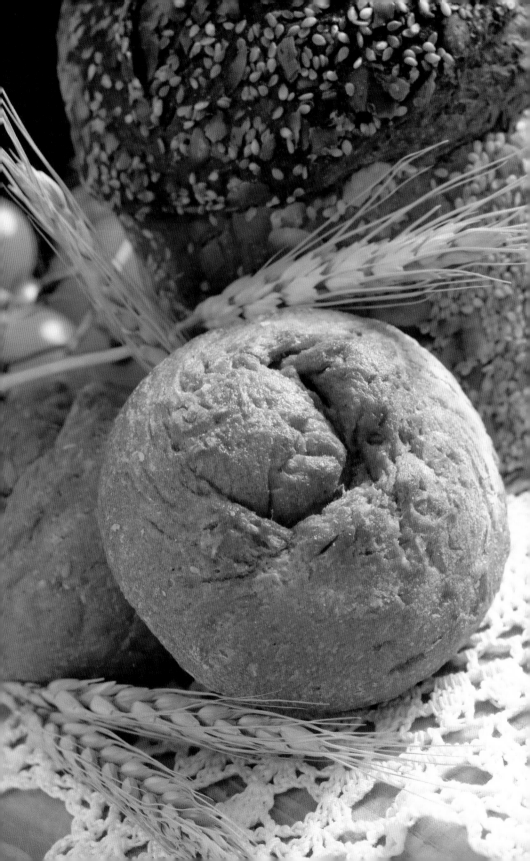

4. Percent of daily value: This column shows the percentage of a particular nutrient that one serving of the food would provide for a person eating 2,000 calories per day. For instance, if the total fat listed is 7 grams, that particular food provides 11 percent of the day's recommended fat allowance. (See no. 5 below for calculation.)

5. Total fats: Most foods contain more than one kind of fat. This number represents the sum total of saturated, polyunsaturated, and monounsaturated fats in the food. There are 4 calories per gram of fat. USDA Food Patterns, the most recent recommendations for food intake, recommends that no more than 30 percent of calories should come from fat, with less than 10 percent coming from saturated fats. This translates to less than 65 grams of fat daily for a person consuming 2,000 calories per day.

6. Saturated fats: Saturated fats are those which are solid at room temperature. They come primarily from animal sources and are associated with heart disease and some forms of cancer. Less than 10 percent of your total calories, or 20 grams, should come from saturated fats.

7. Trans fats: Avoid foods that contain trans fats. Trans fats are chemically altered oils and are present in some stick margarines or shortenings, and many fried and processed foods. They increase serum cholesterol and contribute to heart disease.

8. Polyunsaturated fats: Polyunsaturated fats are found primarily in vegetable oils and include omega-3 and omega-6 fatty acids, which protect the heart.

9. Monounsaturated fats: Monounsaturated fats are also found in vegetable oils, especially canola and olive oil. They increase "good" cholesterol and decrease "bad" cholesterol.

10. Cholesterol: There are two types of cholesterol that contribute to the cholesterol in the blood: HDL or "good" cholesterol and LDL or "bad" cholesterol. Some foods, such as eggs, have been avoided in the past, since they are high in cholesterol. They contain good cholesterol, though, so they don't increase total serum cholesterol or cause heart disease when eaten in moderation.

11. Sodium: For most people, the daily recommended sodium intake is 2,300 milligrams; people who are age fifty or older or who are at risk for high blood pressure should have no more than 1,500 milligrams. It is easy to get too much sodium without even realizing it, so this is a very important number to watch.

12. Total carbohydrates: This number represents the total amount of sugars, starches, sugar alcohols, and fiber in a product. Complex carbohydrates are usually high in fiber and other nutrients. Since fiber doesn't contribute calories, subtract the amount of fiber from the total carbohydrates to get a true picture of the number of carbohydrates a food contains. There are four calories per gram of carbohydrates. USDA Food Patterns recommends that 50 to 65 percent of daily calories (about 300 grams) should come from carbohydrates.

13. Dietary fiber: Aim for 25 to 35 grams of fiber per day. Insoluble fiber helps with digestive processes and soluble fiber decreases "bad" cholesterol. Most Americans only get about half the fiber they need.

14. Sugars: Some sugars occur naturally in fruit, vegetables, dairy products, and other foods. Others are added. Check the ingredients list to see whether sugar, high-fructose corn syrup, or other sweeteners are near the beginning of the list. This indicates that there's a lot of added sugar in a food and it may not be the best choice.

15. Sugar alcohols: Some labels, especially those on sugar-free products, may indicate the amount of sugar alcohol in a product. Look at the ingredients list for names that end in "–ol," such as xylitol, erythritol, mannitol, etc. Sugar alcohols aren't really alcohols at all. Since they are created when plant matter ferments, and the chemical structure looks similar to that of alcohols, they are called sugar alcohols. They have fewer calories than traditional sweeteners and don't affect blood sugar as much. Too much of some sugar alcohols may cause digestive problems.

16. Protein: If a food has more than 9 grams of protein per serving, it's considered a high-protein food. Protein from animal sources contains all of the amino acids that the body can't produce. They are complete proteins. That doesn't mean there aren't other good sources of protein. Complete proteins can also be formed by eating two or more plant-based foods that contain protein together, or by eating a small amount of animal protein with larger amounts of plant-based protein. For example, in Latin cultures, people eat corn tortillas, beans, and rice, which form complete proteins. We should get 10 to 15 percent of our calories from protein. This translates to 45 to 65 grams of protein per day.

17. Nutrients: The label may provide percent daily values for a few nutrients, such as vitamins C and D, calcium, and iron. The daily value is based on a 2,000-calorie diet. Foods that contain 10 to 19 percent of the daily value per serving are considered a "good" source of a nutrient, while those that contain 20 percent or more of the daily value per serving are considered an "excellent" source.

18. Footnote: The footnote at the bottom of the Nutrition Facts label provides the daily values for total fat, saturated fat, cholesterol, sodium, total carbohydrates, and dietary fiber based on 2,000-calorie and 2,500-calorie diets.

19. Ingredients list: The ingredients are listed in order of dominance by weight, so look for foods with healthy ingredients at the beginning of the list. Watch out for ingredients such as beef fat, butter, coconut oil, hydrogenated oils, palm kernel oil, or palm oil, as the product may be too high in saturated fat or contain trans fats. If a product is promoted as "whole grain," check to see if whole grain is listed as the first or second ingredient. The ingredients list can also tell you what kinds of sweeteners are used in the product, such as sugar, honey, high-fructose corn syrup, etc.

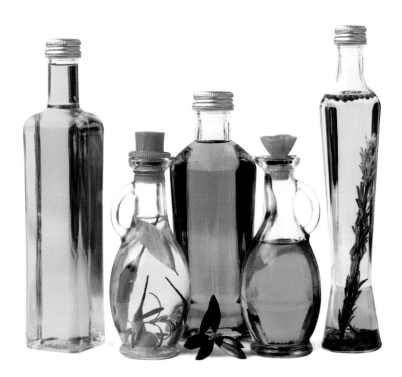

Fat Facts

All fats contain 9 calories per gram, so the calories add up quickly. A tablespoon of any type of fat is 120 calories. A three-ounce lean, broiled hamburger has 14 grams of fat; a restaurant order of Fettucine Alfredo can contain as many as 33 grams of fat and 1,200 calories!

Although my weight-loss regimen recommends two tablespoons of healthy oil per day, I don't go out of my way to add oil to anything. I just make sure to choose healthy fats when I have the option. For example, I use Smart Balance Light on my whole-wheat toast, and canola oil for stir-frying. I eat a salad every day with Newman's Own Lighten Up Low Fat Sesame Ginger Dressing, and I often eat nuts as part of a snack. This way I get the right amount of the right oils from my regular diet.

What are some other ways to cut your fat intake?

- Buy the leanest possible cuts of meat.

- Trim visible fat from meat before cooking.

- When making soup stock, soup, or stew, let it cool in the refrigerator so that the fat floats to the top and hardens. Skim off the hardened fat and reheat soup before serving.

- Experiment with herbs, spices, and flavored vinegars for added flavor so you don't have to resort to butter or cheese.

- Remove the skin from poultry before eating.

- Avoid fried foods, including chicken and shrimp.

- Make buying decisions by reading the Nutrition Facts label to see how much saturated or trans fat a product contains.

- Use a little olive or canola oil instead of butter or lard for cooking.

- Choose fat-free dairy products such as skim milk and fat-free yogurt.

- Forego the bacon bits and cheese on salads, and use reduced-calorie salad dressing. You can pack a lot of fat into a seemingly healthy salad.

- Watch out for cream-based soups and sauces. Instead, make your own by pureeing cooked vegetables with a little broth (see recipe section).

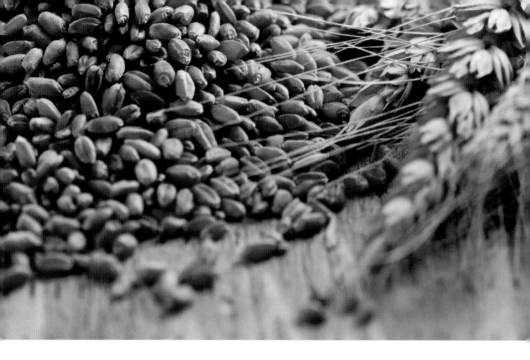

Fiber Up

Getting enough fiber is important to your weight-loss goals. Fiber is present in most plants and provides their support structure. Fiber-rich foods give you that "full" feeling in your stomach, a cue to stop eating. Which takes longer to consume and digest, a cup of apple juice or a whole apple? A slice of white bread or a slice of chewy whole-wheat bread? Which of these makes you feel full longer?

Insoluble fiber, sometimes called "roughage," helps food pass through the digestive tract smoothly, helping to prevent constipation and other bowel problems. It's also thought to help prevent colon cancer. Soluble fiber develops a gel-like consistency in the digestive tract, which binds to fatty acids and promotes their removal. Soluble fiber helps to lower LDL, or "bad," cholesterol levels.

The American Dietetic Association recommends 25 to 35 grams of fiber per day, though the average American only consumes about half of the recommended amount. Good fiber sources are beans, legumes, whole grains such as whole wheat, oats, brown rice, fruits, and vegetables. Processed foods such as white bread or white rice contain very little fiber.

I don't rely on fiber supplements because I want to get fiber from what I eat. Nature has packed nutrients in real foods in the best combinations for the body to use.

If you're raising your fiber intake, do it gradually, and be sure to drink plenty of fluids to avoid stomach distress and/or diarrhea.

Fiber content in foods

Broccoli, cooked	1/2 cup	2.6	grams
Black beans, cooked	1 cup	15	grams
Garbanzo beans, cooked	1 cup	12.5	grams
Sweet corn, cooked	1 cup	3.6	grams
Spinach, cooked	1 cup	4.3	grams
Whole-wheat pasta, cooked	1/2 cup	3.15	grams
Whole-wheat bread	1 slice	4	grams
Raw carrots	1/2 cup	2.5	grams
Lentils, cooked	1/2 cup	7.8	grams
Navel orange	med	3.1	grams
Pear	med	5.5	grams
Zucchini, cooked with skin	1 cup	1.8	grams
Strawberries, sliced	1 cup	2.9	grams
Raspberries	1 cup	8	grams
Sweet potato	1 cup	6.6	grams

Shake the Salt Habit

Too much sodium can cause high blood pressure, stroke, and heart disease. The recommended amount of sodium per day is less than 2,300 milligrams, but most Americans average about 3,400 milligrams of salt per day. It may take time to adjust your taste to less salty foods.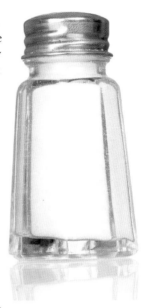

Read Nutrition Facts labels to find the sodium content of foods. Some foods are very high in sodium, especially processed foods, which provide over 70 percent of Americans' sodium intake. For instance, a slice of Tombstone Supreme Pizza has 640 milligrams of sodium. A one-half-cup serving of spicy marinara sauce has 460 milligrams of sodium, and 16 reduced-fat Wheat Thins have 230 milligrams. A four-ounce serving of lean ham contains 1,060 milligrams of sodium, nearly half of your sodium for a whole day. Carbonated beverages, both regular and diet, may also contain sodium. Even if you never use a salt shaker, you may be getting too much sodium. Look for low-sodium options.

When you prepare your own meals, it is easy to control the amount of salt used. I like to use herbs and spices to give my food flavor, and only add salt when absolutely necessary. When eating at restaurants, ask that no salt be added to your meal, or order low-sodium options, if available.

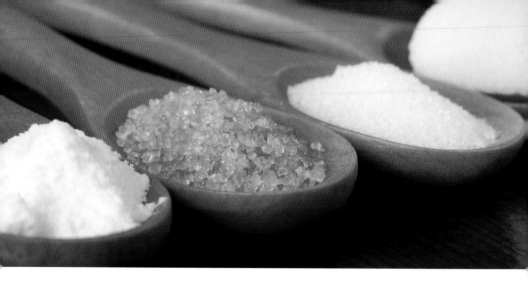

Sugar: The Bittersweet Story

Cookies, candy, doughnuts, gooey desserts, and sweet drinks can be a real temptation. Even though they may say "sugar free," they often contain other ingredients that can sidetrack your weight-loss plan. Additionally, they do not provide your body with the nutrients it needs like the nutrient-dense foods you could be eating. Replace sweetened drinks with water, and grab an orange the next time you are craving sweets.

Treats are hard to live without, so find a healthy substitute. When I gave up my regular habit of malts and milk shakes, I came up with a banana "shake" made from a frozen banana and soy milk, (see recipe on page 193) so I could still have a treat in the evening. I also make a cottage cheese "sundae" using a home-made raspberry sauce poured over one-half cup of nonfat cottage cheese, with a few nuts sprinkled on top. Both of these "treats" keep me satisfied.

Water: A Step in the Right Direction

Water is an often-overlooked nutrient, but it is vitally important. "Getting enough water is crucial if you're trying to lose weight," says Dr. E. Wayne Askew, director of University of Utah's Nutrition Division, in a recent *Deseret News* article. Askew said that not having enough fluid in your body can reduce your resting metabolic rate. This is the amount of calories your body burns while at rest in order to maintain life. Your resting metabolic rate accounts for roughly 60 percent of the calories burned by the body, so you definitely don't want it slowing down!

Getting enough fluids is also crucial if you're stepping up your exercise program. Being dehydrated reduces muscular endurance and physical work capacity. This is why athletes are always striving to stay hydrated during competition.

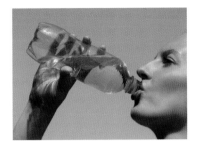

Water also regulates body temperature, carries nutrients and oxygen to cells, carries waste out of the body, and cushions and protects joints and organs.

Water is lost though urine, sweat, and respiration. The brain's thirst center lags behind water loss. By the time you feel thirsty, you're already a bit dehydrated, so keep a bottle of water handy—and use it!

Some people say that when they feel hungry, they drink a big glass of water. Often they realize they were really thirsty, not hungry.

Drinking water before a meal is a good idea, according to a study done at Virginia Tech. When middle-aged and older adults drank two cups of water before each meal, they consumed between 75 and 90 fewer calories at the meal, and eventually lost more weight than those who skipped drinking water. Eight glasses of water is the standard daily recommendation.

When running errands, I take a filled one-quart water bottle with me, and I also stash one in a cooler that I keep in my car. I find that I can easily drink a pint of water while I'm out and about.

Often I'll drink warm water before eating dinner to avoid overeating, just like the Chinese do. They believe cold drinks cool down your system, and then it has to be warmed up again. When I travel in foreign countries, I drink bottled water, but at home I drink filtered tap water.

The least expensive and most effective way to keep up your fluids is by drinking water. Flavored sports drinks containing sodium aren't necessary if you're exercising fewer than three hours, and most of them are high in calories. If you're trying to lose weight, pure water is always the best choice.

Don't Drink Your Calories

Soda pop, fruit-flavored drinks, sports drinks, and other sweet beverages all pack on unnecessary pounds. Americans consume 300 more calories a day in sugary beverages than they did thirty years ago, according to Barry Popkin, director of the University of North Carolina Nutrition Obesity Research Center. His research has shown that people who drink water instead of sugary drinks tend to eat more fruits and vegetables and consume fewer calories throughout the day.

The USDA's 2010 Dietary Guidelines for Americans concurs, adding that people who drink more sugar-sweetened beverages have higher body weight compared to those who drink less.

Depending on the brand, a 12-ounce can of sweetened soda contains 140 to 170 calories. That's just about as much as one of my daily snacks and is not nearly as satisfying!

- Beware of healthy-sounding fruit-flavored drinks, which are mainly water and sweetener. An eight-ounce cup of Sunny Delight, for instance, contains 130 calories.

- Look for the term "100 percent fruit juice." The label may say "made with real juice," but the actual "real juice" content found in the small print may be only 5 to 10 percent. If you consume fruit-flavored drinks instead of juice, you're missing out on important nutrients that come from fruit.

- Even so, real juice is high in calories as well (orange juice is 110 calories per 8-ounce cup). You're better off eating that whole orange; you get all the same nutrients, plus fiber, which will help you feel more satisfied.

- Avoid caffeinated sodas and "energy drinks," since most of them are high in sugar and caffeine. They're a poor substitute for proper rest and nutrition.

Got Dairy?

Dairy products contribute many nutrients for good health, such as calcium, vitamin D, and potassium, and are linked to strong bones and effective weight loss. The 2010 Dietary Guidelines for Americans recommends three cups per day of fat-free or low-fat dairy products because they provide the same nutrients with less fat and fewer calories. Skim milk is 86 calories per cup, with 4 calories coming from fat. One percent milk is 110 calories, with 20 coming from fat. Low-fat, or 2 percent milk, is 120 to 130 calories per cup, with 45 of those calories from fat. That's a hefty increase in fat.

If you don't like milk or if it gives you digestive problems, there are several good substitutes, including soy, almond, and rice milk.

Jackie suggests I limit my intake of cheese to one serving per day because it has a high concentration of fat. I choose reduced-fat cheese or hard cheese when possible. Here are a few of the ways I use cheese to complement the flavor of my healthy food choices:

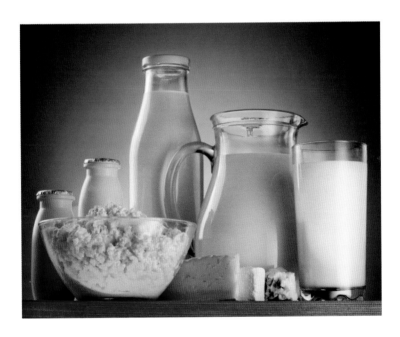

Hard cheese: Parmigiano Reggiano comes both grated and in hard blocks which I shred so that a little goes a long way. I also like to use this cheese on spring greens with a little light salad dressing. This cheese pops the flavor of soups, butternut squash, and spaghetti. Be sure to portion it so you stay within your calorie limit, but explore the flavor possibilities. Check the deli counter at your supermarket for this and other flavorful hard cheeses.

Light string cheese: At 80 calories per stick, light string cheese is great for snacks. I use a combination of carbohydrate, fat, and protein for each of my snacks, and string cheese gives me both fat and protein. When I add a piece of fruit, I have the perfect snack for keeping up my energy mid-morning, mid-afternoon, or early evening.

Laughing Cow Light Creamy Swiss: When I want a spreadable cheese, I use this one. At only 35 calories per wedge, it can be spread on a slice of whole-wheat bread for a satisfying snack, and it's highly flavorful. One downside to these small pieces of cheese is that the sodium content is high. One serving contains 220 mg, or 9 percent of your daily intake.

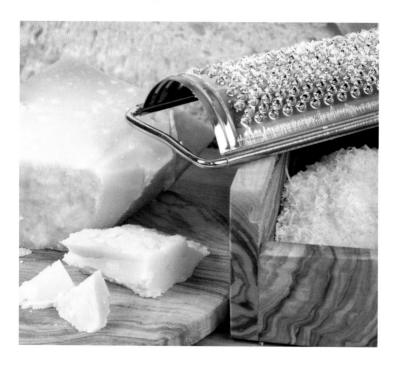

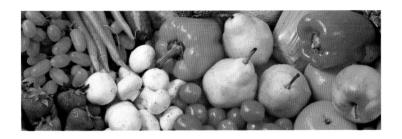

Power-Load with Fruits and Vegetables

Once you start feeding yourself high-performance foods, it won't be long until you're power-loading your meals with produce. Increasing your intake of fruits and vegetables is one of the best ways to add nutrients to your diet. Fruits and vegetables are high in vitamins, minerals, and antioxidants. They also contain fiber that helps in digestion and works with the body to move food though the system. Most fruits and vegetables are also low in calories. It's the fancy dips, or the cheese and butter sauces that you add to them, which raise the calorie count.

Fruits and vegetables also add variety and color to your meals. Without them, you'd be stuck with the browns and whites of meats, grains, and dairy. There would be no bright green broccoli, vivid orange carrots, or crimson tomatoes. Think of the rainbow when selecting fruits and vegetables: choose a palette of color to maximize flavor and nutrition. The pigments that give fruit and vegetables their bright colors are actually nutrients. For instance, bright orange and yellow foods, such as carrots, mangoes, and squash, contain beta-carotene. Tomatoes, watermelon, and other red fruits contain lycopene, shown to reduce the risk of prostate cancer. Blackberries, blueberries, and raspberries contain anthocyanids, which help prevent heart disease; raspberries and strawberries contain ellagic acid, a powerful cancer preventative. Even natural fiber that gives plants their shape is good for you, helping to eliminate body waste and promoting colon health. Eating fruits and vegetables really is the best way to power-load your body for weight-loss success.

Fun fact: Many vegetables tend to look like the parts of the body they help the most. Look at the cross section of a carrot and it resembles an eye; Brussels sprouts on the cane look like a spinal column, and they're good for nerve conduction. The inside of a tomato is chambered similar to the heart.

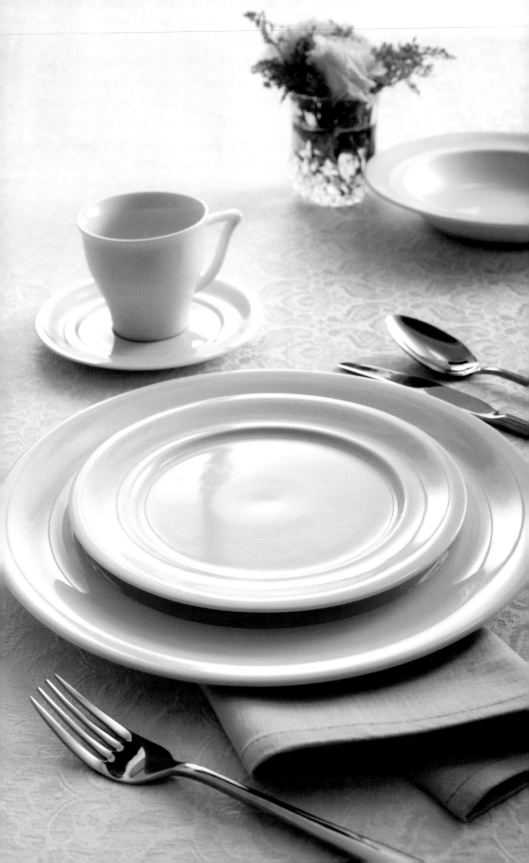

Chapter 5
Strategies

Keeping Evening Eating Under Control

For most American families, dinner is the main meal. Everyone is busy during the day, so there is more time in the evening to fix a balanced dinner, eat together, and relax. But if you haven't planned a healthy meal in advance, it's easy to grab whatever is handy and make poor food choices. Then comes evening TV watching and the desire to nibble a little more, picking up extra calories. My dinners now consist of a green salad, three ounces of protein, and two or three vegetables. Occasionally I'll add a whole-grain starch, such as whole-wheat bread, whole-wheat pasta, or brown rice.

Here are some ideas for keeping calories down in the evening:

1. Nibbling while preparing food: It's possible for people to consume a whole meal just by tasting and nibbling before they ever sit down to the dinner table. Chewing sugar-free gum while I prepare a meal makes me think twice about tasting the food. To taste for flavor while cooking, just dip a spoon in the pot and sample only what clings to the spoon.

2. Cleaning up after dinner: A common habit is to finish off anything left on a plate or in a serving dish while cleaning up. Make a commitment to yourself not to nibble on anything after you have finished your meal. Perhaps you can assign family members to take turns with the clean-up. Remember the saying, "It's better for extra food to go to waste than to add inches to your waist." You can always try the gum trick here, too.

3. After-dinner eating: After finishing dinner, I would often sit in my kitchen watching television, thinking about what I could eat next. This is the time I would bring out the ice cream, and I very seldom stopped with a small scoop. So I kicked the TV out of the kitchen and began to plan urgent tasks elsewhere, taking my mind off eating. Many times we eat because we are bored, not because we are hungry.

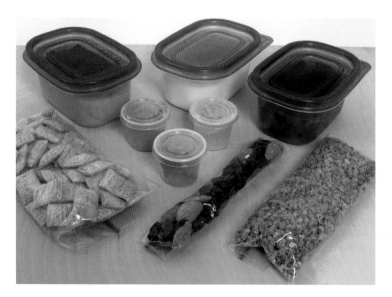

Portion Control

How often do you find yourself enjoying some cookies, or maybe potato chips, only to find that you've eaten the whole bag? I remember when I used to sit down to eat one tablespoon of reduced-calorie peanut butter. Fifteen tablespoons later I would decide I should quit! Learning appropriate portion sizes, measuring them out, and sticking to my plan were key to changing my eating patterns. Measuring portions helps put boundaries on what you can eat. I notice when I eat from a large bowl or an open container, I seem to have a chip in my brain that says I can go back for "just a little" more. When the food is measured out, my brain chip says, "You must stop; you have had your serving."

Nutrition Facts

Serving Size 1/2 cup slices (85.0 g)

Amount Per Serving

Calories 37	Calories from Fat 1
	% Daily Value
Total Fat 0.2g	**0%**
Saturated Fat 0.0g	**0%**
Polyunsaturated Fat 0.1g	
Monounsaturated Fat 0.0g	
Cholesterol 0mg	**0%**
Sodium 65mg	**3%**
Total Carbohydrates 8.5g	**3%**
Dietary Fiber 1.7g	**7%**
Sugars 6.8g	
Protein 1.4g	
Vitamin A 1% •	Vitamin C 5%
Calcium 1% •	Iron 4%

* Based on a 2000 calorie diet

See more extended nutritional details

Remember to check the Nutrition Facts label on the back of every food package. The serving size will be given by measure and weight, so you can either use measuring equipment or a scale to divide portions. Fresh ingredients don't have nutrition labels, but you can find all the information you need online. The USDA has a searchable database at http://www.nal.usda.gov/fnic/foodcomp/search/ where you can find serving sizes, calorie count, and thousands of food items.

Tools for portion control:

1. Measuring cups and spoons.

2. Scales.
An adequate kitchen scale shouldn't cost any more than $30, although you can spend a lot more than that. It should be fairly accurate and convertible between grams and ounces. Mine has a feature which allows me to place the container on the scale then push "0." Then I'm only weighing the food and not the container. Scales are available online or in local kitchen and hardware supply stores (see page 134).

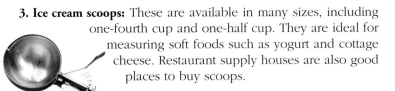

3. Ice cream scoops:
These are available in many sizes, including one-fourth cup and one-half cup. They are ideal for measuring soft foods such as yogurt and cottage cheese. Restaurant supply houses are also good places to buy scoops.

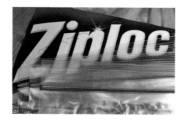

Containers for portion control:

1. Ziploc® sandwich bags: I often use sandwich bags to portion out my snacks and four-ounce cuts of meat or other protein, which I buy in bulk.

2. Plastic containers with lids: These are available in several sizes, but the size I use most holds one cup.

3. Single-serving cups with lids: I buy these in packages of 100 from a local restaurant supply store. You can also order them online from restaurant suppliers. I measure one tablespoon of reduced-fat peanut butter into these.

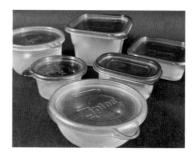

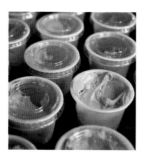

4. Glass bottle: I also bought this glass bottle at a restaurant supply store, and I fill it with oil to keep handy beside my stove—quick and easy!

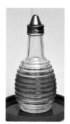

Here are some of the foods that I premeasure and the portion sizes I use:

Food	Preparation	Portion	Container	Storage
lean meats	uncooked	4 oz	Ziploc bag	freezer
fat-free yogurt		8 oz	1-cup container	refrigerator
nonfat cottage cheese		4 oz	½-cup container	refrigerator
butternut squash	precooked	8 oz	1-cup container	refrigerator
blueberries		8 oz	1-cup container	refrigerator

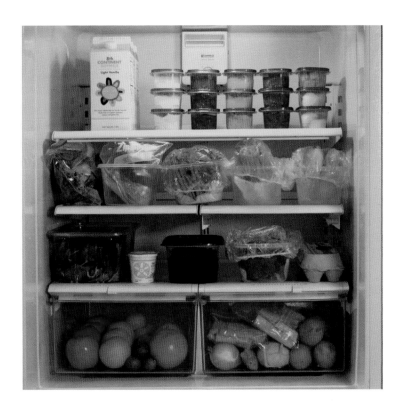

When my refrigerator is loaded and ready for the week, it looks like this. On the top shelves you can see containers of yogurt, cottage cheese, squash, and salsa.

According to the USDA's 2010 Dietary Guidelines for Americans:

- A serving of meat is 4 ounces raw and 3 ounces cooked, or about the size of a deck of cards. Serving sizes for other proteins would be ½ cup of beans or two eggs.

- A serving of grains is equal to one slice of whole-grain bread, one-half whole-wheat bagel, a small muffin, one-half cup cooked pasta or rice, two four-inch pancakes, or one six-inch tortilla.

- A serving of fruit or vegetables is about one-half cup or one medium-sized fruit.

- A serving of skim milk or nonfat yogurt is one cup, nonfat cottage cheese one-half cup, and hard cheese one ounce.

Here are some quick portion-control guides:

- A medium-sized piece of fruit is the size of a hard ball.
- 1 ounce of cheese is about the size of four stacked dice.
- 1 ounce of nuts should fit into the palm of your hand.
- 1 teaspoon of margarine or butter is about the size of a thumb tip.

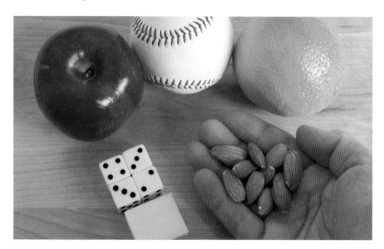

Put Your Meals on Autopilot

The National Weight Control Register, which tracks people who successfully lost an average of 70 pounds and kept it off for more than a year, says one of the keys to losing and keeping weight off is to develop "autopilot meals."

In the long run, it's not a diet that will take you to success. It is developing a workable food plan that will support you. I developed my meal plans around the healthy foods I enjoy, and Jackie helped me determine the portion sizes that would help me lose the most weight.

I develop a meal plan each week. After grocery shopping, I prepare and portion in advance, so it's easy and convenient to stay on my program.

As you create meals that contain all the basics, including a protein, complex carbohydrate, lots of vegetables, and a little fat, write them down and prepare them often. Soon you'll develop more meals that will help you lose and maintain weight.

Challenges and Solutions

If you are going to keep the weight off, you will have to find solutions that work for you. You can't rely on a quick-fix, short-term diet; I am always learning new techniques to support my weight loss. As I share my challenges with Jackie, she supports me in finding solutions.

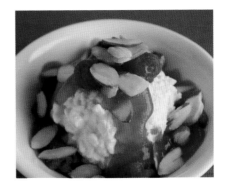

My ability to face the challenges gets easier with every success. I have accepted the fact that many foods, such as milk shakes, fries, and doughnuts, are not on my approved eating list anymore.

Sports teams always identify challenges and then plan strategies to help them win. They map them out and practice over and over to develop the skills they need to be winners. This is the same process I have followed to lose weight.

Here are a few of the challenges and solutions that keep me in the losing game.

1. Family birthday parties: When my extended family gets together for a birthday party, there's always cake and ice cream. Neither is on my food plan, so I'll spoon fruit over cottage cheese instead. Occasionally, if the ice cream is homemade or extra-special, I'll have a spoonful. I have gotten to the point where I am just as satisfied with my cottage cheese and fruit as I would have been with cake and ice cream.

In fact, my newest concoction is a cottage cheese "sundae." I have whipped up some delectable ones using the fresh fruit I buy at farmers' markets. My favorite is a sauce made from unsweetened raspberries. I put one-half cup of nonfat cottage cheese in a lidded plastic container that I can take with me. Then I pour one-half cup of the sauce on top and add one tablespoon of slivered or chopped almonds. The total calories are under 200, and I feel completely satisfied after eating it. (See page 195 for a sundae variation.)

2. Group eating events: These include potluck dinners, office parties, and meetings where snacks are on hand. First, I try to find out in advance what will be served, and then I put an alternate plan in place. For a long time I belonged to an organization that served pizza at a monthly event. Every time I attended I packed a healthy dinner, usually a salmon sandwich, with fruit and vegetables on the side, in a small cooler. People would walk by and say, "I sure wish I had that for dinner."

Recently I was invited to a luau, so I took a cooler packed with my own minimeal. As I went through the buffet line, I selected three ounces of cooked pork then opened my bag and added a few healthy extras. All my friends know how hard I'm working at reducing my weight, and they are very supportive when I am invited to their homes to eat.

3. The temptation to stop for ice cream: This used to be a favorite pastime of mine. I would drive by my local ice cream shop and it would seem to say, "Dian, I have a wonderful shake waiting for you." Since that's off-limits for me now, I found a replacement, my frozen banana "smoothie" (see recipe on page 193).

4. Energy drop while running errands: While running errands, I used to whip into McDonald's and pick up a cheeseburger for a dollar. Sometimes I even had more than one. No more. Now I pack a car snack kit with bottled water and several 150-calorie snacks. That way when I have an energy drop, I reach into my small cooler and grab a bag. My energy level is soon back to normal, without the guilt or the calories.

I use Ziploc sandwich bags to store snacks, and I always pack snacks that are nonperishable. Taking snacks with me also keeps me from having an all-blowout-meal as soon as I get home.

Remember, it's not about dieting; it's about changing the way you deal with food. Even small steps like these make a big difference.

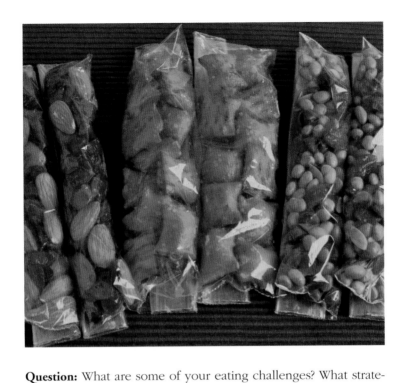

Question: What are some of your eating challenges? What strategies can you use?

_____

_____

_____

_____

_____

_____

_____

_____

_____

_____

_____

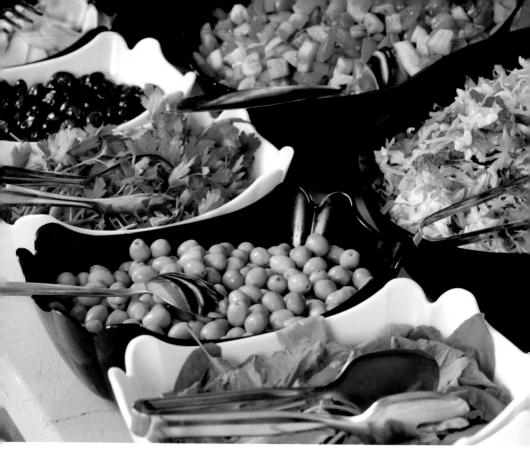

Set Yourself Up for Success When Eating Out

Choosing the right foods when I eat out, or when I'm on vacation, can be difficult, especially if I'm unfamiliar with the area. The food is rarely what I would fix for myself at home, and I'm often tempted to order something that's not good for my weight-loss program. Another challenge can be recognizing all the ingredients and guessing their amounts and calorie counts in a particular dish. How much oil does this salad dressing contain? Do they use lean cuts of meat?

Planning a strategy ahead of time sets you up for success. A helpful Web site to visit before eating away from home is http://www.healthydiningfinder.com/. This site provides examples of healthy dishes you might find at local restaurants, along with calorie counts and nutritional information.

How can you master the art of eating out while maintaining control?

1. Decide what you want to order before you get to the restaurant. I often go to a restaurant's Web site beforehand. Many of the chains will list the calorie count for each dish on the menu. I remember going out with friends and all of us ordering a delicious salad because we thought the calories would be minimal. I came home, checked the restaurant's Web site, and discovered the salad we thought was a winner had more than 850 calories!

2. When attending a business lunch or impromptu event, order a grilled chicken salad. I prefer low-calorie, high-flavor dressings, so I bring my own, usually Newman's Own Lighten Up Low Fat Sesame Ginger Dressing. Grilled fish with a double order of vegetables (no butter) is also another safe choice.

3. Say no to rolls, bread, and chips that precede the meal. They're dangerous because you tend to fill up on empty calories.

4. Keep a few restaurants in mind where you know you can find good choices. When people ask me where I would like to go, I usually suggest a particular Mexican grill where the food is fresh, delicious, and nutritious.

5. Watch out for "portion distortion." Restaurant portions can be two or three times bigger than standard. There's that urge to finish everything on your plate because it's just sitting there, and it seems a shame to waste it. Ask for a take-home box as soon as your meal arrives. Then quickly box up half of the meal so that it's out of sight and take it home for tomorrow's lunch.

6. Don't surrender to the buffet. Eating at a buffet can be dangerous, but if you prepare in advance, you can avoid calorie overload. If my friends suggest a buffet, I recommend we go to one that serves soup and salad. If not, I eat the fresh salad items with my own salad dressing, vegetables, and three ounces (cooked) of protein for the main course. If I forget the dressing, I use a light house dressing, lemon juice, or vinegar and olive oil.

7. Dessert is my kryptonite. It's hard to sit and watch my friends "ooh" and "aah" about their dessert. Most restaurants have some type of fresh fruit on hand. I take a carton of yogurt and ask them to bring the fruit to me in a bowl. For example, a banana with yogurt keeps me from feeling deprived.

8. Find someone to whom you can be accountable. E-mail or call your support person, and review goals and strategies before dining out. Writing them down and talking to someone gives you reinforcement.

Questions: What are some of your challenges when you're eating out? What are some strategies for handling them?

_____

_____

_____

_____

_____

_____

_____

_____

Question: What are some of your favorite restaurants where you know you can get healthy choices?

_____

_____

_____

_____

_____

_____

_____

_____

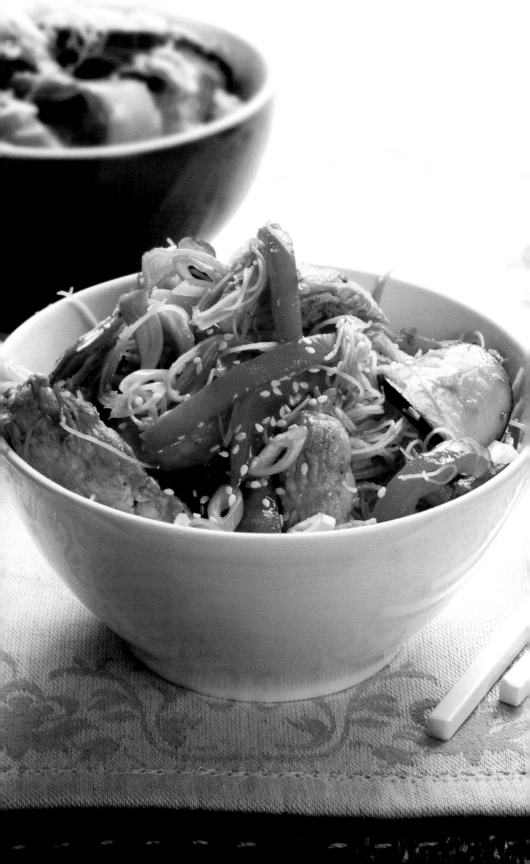

Set Up Your Car to Serve Fast Food

At my heaviest weight, I would frequent fast-food outlets while running errands. It was one of the chief ways I packed on the pounds. No more fast food on the road for me!

I now have a "fast-food restaurant" in my car, equipped to fill me up, whether it is a quick snack or a light meal. All I have to do is pull off the road and open my cooler filled with pre-portioned, healthy "fast food" designed for my now-leaner body. You can also set this up to satisfy hungry kids when you're out running errands or on road trips.

A favorite fast-food snack is 10 almonds and 2 tablespoons of raisins. For a light meal, I have a small can of salmon (don't forget a small can opener) and 10 whole-wheat Triscuits, which give me a little more energy.

To set up fast food in your car, use a container that will fit snugly without sliding around in the car interior or trunk. Then make a list of combinations of healthy, nonperishable foods you can eat on the go.

Next, portion your food into individual packages so they're quick and easy to pull out and eat. Otherwise, you could have a "blowout" and consume the whole bag. Ziploc sandwich bags work well to hold about 150 calories per snack. Even though the bags can hold more, I limit the contents to the portion size I need. Just think of the money you will save and health benefits you will enjoy in your own "fast-food restaurant."

Question: What are some healthy foods you could pack in your car for on-the-go snacks?

_____

_____

_____

_____

_____

_____

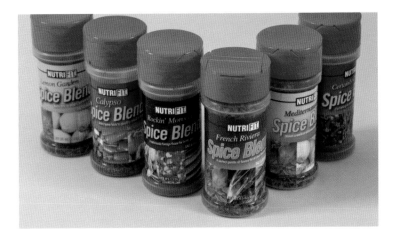

Favorite Food Products

Any calorie counter's biggest challenge is finding delicious but low-calorie foods. Here are a few that have been a welcome addition to my eating plan.

NutriFit Spice Blends: These spice blends contain no salt or sugar. There are six different spice blends designed to flavor everything from salads, soups, dips, and meats to desserts (www.nutrifit online.com).

Ultra Gel®: This instant starch thickens liquids without cooking. It gives homemade salad dressings body without adding many calories and thickens fat-free broths into deliciously "legal" soups and sauces. (See the following Web site: www.cornabys.com/about_us.html.)

Reduced-Fat Peanut Butter: This tastes the same as regular peanut butter. All they do is remove a little oil from the peanuts, which brings down the calorie count without affecting the taste.

Miracle Whip Fat-Free Dressing: If you like the flavor of Miracle Whip, you will like this product. There are only 15 calories in one tablespoon. I use it mainly to moisten egg salad and salmon for sandwiches.

Newman's Own® Lighten Up Low Fat Sesame Ginger Dressing: My favorite for salads and vegetables, with only 35 calories in two tablespoons. Some salad dressings contain as many as 150 calories for the same amount. When I eat out, I often take this dressing with me in a small bottle. It does have a lot of sodium so I watch my portion size.

Smart Balance® Light: This light spread is a flavorful blend of oils, including olive oil and flaxseed oil. It contains 50 calories per tablespoon, compared with 120 calories in butter or margarine.

8th Continent® Soy Milk Light Vanilla: I would never have switched to a soy milk had I not been allergic to milk, but I find the flavor of this, at 60 calories per cup, even better than skim milk, which is 100 calories.

Ezekiel 4:9® Cereals: A half-cup portion of this blend of grains provides a complete protein, which you don't get when you eat one-grain cereals. It is very filling, and I rarely feel hungry an hour after I have eaten it. You can buy this at a health and nutrition store.

Kirkland Signature® Canned Salmon: This salmon makes a wonderful quick and easy sandwich spread, which I take as my traveling lunch. Since airlines provide few food options on flights nowadays, this sandwich, with a few fresh vegetables, makes a perfect portable lunch.

Cornaby® 10-Calorie Spreadable Fruit: This fruit spread tastes delicious on whole-wheat toast or stirred into unflavored yogurt. It is sugar-free and contains about 85 percent fruit, while traditional jams are 65 percent sugar. With only 10 calories per tablespoon and lots of fresh flavors, I can afford to splurge. (See the following Web site: www.cornabys.com/about_us.)

Question: What are some food products that will help you with your weight-loss goals?

_____

_____

_____

_____

_____

_____

_____

Key Tools

Through the years I have found some key tools to support me in losing and maintaining weight. Here are some that I use regularly.

Pedometer: Moving is vital to healthy weight loss. A year or so ago I decided I needed to know how many daily steps I was taking in order to augment my exercise. I wanted a particular kind of pedometer, so I read reviews on Amazon.com. After consulting _Consumer Guide_, I found one for under $30—an Omron HJ-112N. I keep it in my pocket and use a small fastener to attach it to my slacks. Off I go.

On an average day in the office, I walk approximately two miles (5,000 steps). To maintain weight, you should walk 10,000 steps a day; to lose weight, increase that to 12,000 or more. Checking my pedometer throughout the day pushes me to walk more. It also keeps a record of my steps for seven days.

Food scales: Portion control was, and still is, a challenge, so a food scale is a must for preparing proper portion sizes. I prefer a scale that measures both ounces and grams. My Weight Watchers® scale allows me to zero out the scale after I've placed an empty container on it so I am weighing my ingredients and not the container. After I add the first ingredient, I can zero out the scale again and weigh another ingredient in the container. I find that after a few times doing this, I know the right amount of each item to put in without having to weigh it.

Some of the foods that I weigh are cheese, salad dressings, meats, and reduced-calorie peanut butter.

Ziploc sandwich bags: Premeasured items require containers of various sizes. I use the bags to portion meats, snacks, and breakfast cereals.

Plastic containers: Several companies manufacture sturdy, inexpensive, long-lasting containers that are approved for food. Keep three or four sizes on hand.

One-cup sizes are ideal for measuring yogurt, cottage cheese, and cooked vegetables. Larger containers are excellent for storing fruits, vegetables, and other items for later use.

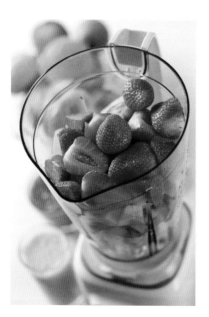

Blender: Every night I look foward to my frozen banana shake. When I attend a gathering where candy and cookies are served, I just kept telling myself, "I am not eating these empty calories! I am going home to my tasty, healthy banana shake."

Double boiler: I use a double boiler once or twice a day for steaming vegetables.

Cast-iron wok: I use my cast-iron wok all the time because it holds the heat well and keeps the food in the center of the pan for even cooking.

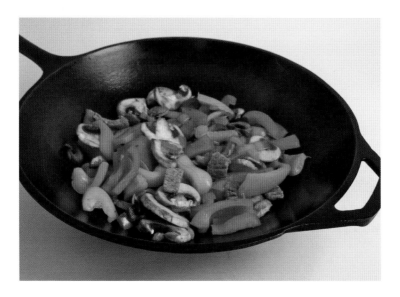

Question: What are some tools that can help with your weight-loss goals?

_____

_____

_____

_____

_____

_____

_____

_____

_____

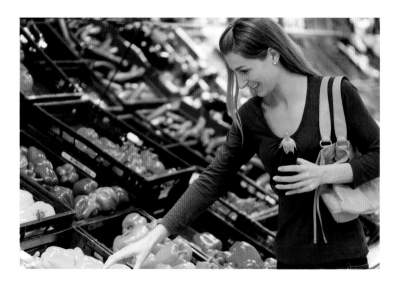

Shopping Tips

The foods you bring home from the store and put into your cupboard directly affect your health. When I began losing weight, one of my first "Jackie" assignments was to clear my cupboards of all the foods I shouldn't eat. Next was to purchase the right kinds of foods, bring them home, and organize them.

Plan your menu for the week, and then make a market order. When you shop with this in hand, you are less likely to buy impulse items. To make a market order, fold an 8½ by 11-inch sheet into thirds vertically (from the top to the bottom of the paper), and then in thirds again horizontally (from side to side of the paper), making nine squares to write in. Starting with the top squares write "produce," "dairy," and "meat." In the middle squares write "frozen," "canned," and "dry goods." Across the bottom squares go "household supplies," "miscellaneous," and "other errands." Under each heading I list everything I need (see page 206).

Check the newspaper or Internet for sales on produce and other grocery items. This will save money as well as calories. At the store, shop the fresh produce aisle, then meat, dairy, cereal, bread, etc. Try to buy the most nutrient-dense foods with the least amount of added sodium, and check labels to make sure they fall into your prescribed program. Wherever possible, avoid processed foods.

I watch for sales on lean meat and buy in quantity. At home I cut it into individual portions and freeze, thawing in the refrigerator a few days before using it.

Whole-wheat bread, which I also buy in quantity and on sale, freezes well. I save about 50 percent on both my meats and breads. I usually pass on foods without labels, except meat or produce, as the sugar, fat, and salt content are unknown.

One of my favorite activities is visiting farmers' markets during the summer and fall. The only way I could have fresher food is to have grown it in my own garden. I enjoy meeting the farmers who have nurtured the crops and asking them questions about their produce. Each time I go, I bring home new techniques for preparing and storing my purchases. If you don't have farmers' markets in your area, look for roadside produce stands or locally grown produce in your favorite supermarket.

Refrigerator: "Set Up for Weight Loss"

When you order a meal in a restaurant, you expect a wait of fifteen to twenty minutes. When I began a serious weight-loss plan, I knew I would have to work the same kind of turn-around time into my meal preparation or I would not stick to my new eating habits.

I worked on my system over a weekend when I had time to try different setups. I loved eating at restaurants where I could see the chef cooking and observed that when an order for a dish came in, the ingredients he or she needed were already prepped and ready to go. In a similar way, I reorganized my refrigerator so that I could look inside, get inspired for what I wanted to cook, and whip up a delicious, nutritious meal in just fifteen minutes.

Here is my set-up:

Top shelf: Soy milk is to one side. The back is stacked with one-cup containers filled with premeasured, ready-to-go snacks and side dishes. You'll find one-half-cup portions of nonfat cottage cheese, one-cup portions of nonfat yogurt, butternut squash, salsa, etc. On the top shelf there is also a four-ounce package of meat thawing until ready to use.

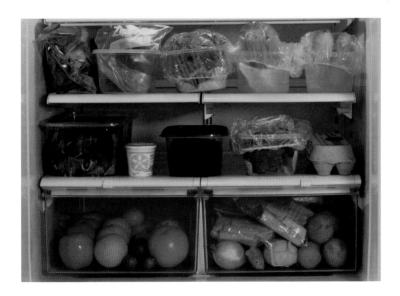

The next two shelves: Vegetables are the mainstay of my diet, so the contents of the next two shelves contain the backbone of my eating program. Several rectangular plastic containers, all the same size, are lined with a paper towel (towels absorb excess moisture to prolong the shelf life of produce) and filled with various vegetables. Some that you'll find in my fridge today are celery, green beans, mushrooms, peppers, and Brussels sprouts. Each container has a plastic shower-cap-type lid, which you can buy in most supermarkets.

The next shelf down holds mixed spring greens that I buy every week for my daily green salad.

In the two bottom drawers are the fruits and vegetables I use in smaller amounts, such as onions, sweet potatoes, and carrots.

In the fridge door you will find nonfat Miracle Whip, dressings, grated hard cheese, Smart Balance Light spread, and nonfat cream cheese.

All I have to do when I want to fix a meal is open the refrigerator door, select the meats and vegetables, and prepare them.

Taking time to design a system that works for you will allow you to produce a healthy meal faster (and cheaper) than patronizing either a fast-food outlet or restaurant.

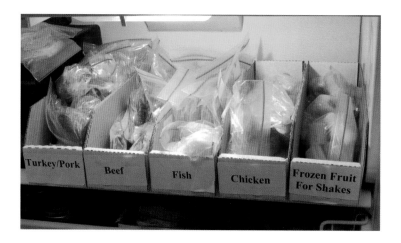

Freezer: My Weight-Loss Must

The freezer has been an economical tool, making it possible to take advantage of sales, to set up my portion sizes for meals, and to freeze them until ready for use. There are also several entrees, such as chili, that I make in batches and freeze for later use.

Not long ago I visited my local meat market for ground pork. The pork on display was much too fatty, so I shared my dissatisfaction with the butcher. He mentioned a sale on sirloin pork and said, "It's very lean, and if you would like, I will grind that up for you." I saved $1.60 per pound by buying 10 pounds which he wrapped in one-pound packages for freezing. I also bought 10 pounds of lean sirloin steaks which I cut into four-ounce portions, stored in Ziploc bags, and froze.

I will often buy two roasted chickens—one to eat during the week and one to portion into three-ounce servings and freeze. I always keep several servings of turkey patties on hand, as well as lean steaks, pork loin, and two or three types of fish.

I keep several small boxes in the freezer, where I store my meat and frozen fruits for easy retrieval. The boxes are labeled "Turkey/Pork," "Beef," "Fish" "Chicken," and "Frozen Fruit For Shakes."

Every third day I remove the frozen packages of meat I plan to use in the next few days and place them in plastic containers in the refrigerator to slowly thaw, which usually takes a day or two.

Another frozen favorite is corn (from the farmer's market). I blanch it, cut it from the cob, and freeze it. I also roast tomatoes, onion, and garlic, drop them into the blender, then let the puree simmer on the stove until reduced. The sauce is then ready for quart-size freezer bags or jars. (See Light and Lean Tomato Sauce on page 197.)

This Web site offers additional details about freezing: http://ohioline.osu.edu/hyg-fact/5000/pdf/5402.pdf.

Set up your freezer to work for you.

Professionals Are Important to the Weight-Loss Process

Since I was more than 125 pounds overweight, I had debilitating physical complications to recover from. I had been morbidly obese for over ten years, which put stress on my muscles, bones, and heart; the cartilage in my right knee was mostly gone and had been for years. My doctor once told me if I would lose 100 pounds I would think I had a new knee. He also told me to put off having knee surgery for as long as I could. The problem with my knee is what led me to decide I had to do whatever I could to lose weight.

A friend and I had lunch in a restaurant on the top floor of the Joseph Smith Memorial Building in downtown Salt Lake City. I was in so much pain that I took my mother's walker in the event I couldn't walk on my own. When my friend saw my condition, she said, "I have a chiropractor who can help you." I resisted, as I had already tried one and had not received much help.

A few days later she called to say she had set me up to see Dr. Bruce Nielson, the chiropractor for the Utah Jazz. He had a unique approach. He had a massage therapist, Walt Oder, break down the scar tissue, a very painful process, before Dr. Nielson worked on my knee. He would then perform various treatments to help stabilize and heal it. Through weight loss and these treatments, I have been able to indefinitely postpone major knee surgery and now have very little pain.

The next step was the recovery of my muscles. Knowing I would need help getting back into condition, I joined the Salt Lake County Recreation program engaging in water aerobics and lifting weights. In the weight room, I was not sure where to start, so Jackie Keller suggested that the next time I was in Los Angeles, I should stop by and work with her trainer, Rick Barke.

Rick took me through some routines designed to build my muscles, which had been very weakened for years. The strength training was basic, but helped me boost my metabolism. Each workout began with a five-minute warm-up walk around the track. He gave me rou-

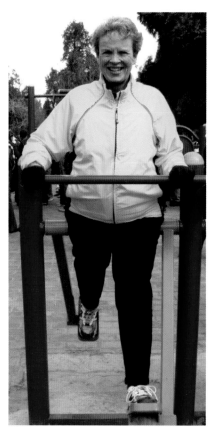

Exercising in China

tines for each part of my body—back, stomach, arms, and legs—specially designed for me. A certified trainer can be very helpful in evaluating where you are and developing a muscle-strengthening program for you.

At 300-plus pounds, I felt too huge to be going to the weight room, and I often had to tell myself, "What other people think about me is none of my business."

I stopped on a recent layover in Los Angeles, and Rick was very excited to see the progress I had made. Then he said, "You must keep active the rest of your life—just keep moving."

Professionals can be great supports as you begin a life change that can seem daunting and even impossible at times.

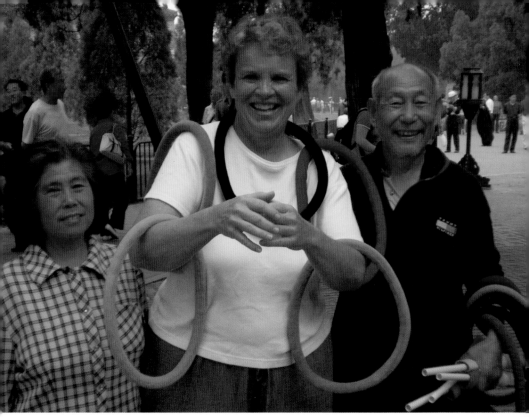

Chinese friends present me with Olympic rings at the Temple of Heaven in Beijing, 2008.

Choosing the Right Doctor

An often-overlooked piece of an effective weight-loss program is determining whether there is illness or imbalance that might interfere with your body's ability to efficiently burn calories and absorb the vital nutrients provided through a healthy eating plan. It is well known that there are conditions that might affect your metabolism and even prevent the loss of weight regardless of exercise and a healthy diet.

It is important that you find a physician who is trained and committed to your overall health by performing a thorough assessment of your physical health and body chemistry. With his or her support, you can optimize your weight loss and put yourself on a path to even greater health. A comprehensive approach to your overall health that includes exercise, good nutrition, and illness prevention is vital to a lean and healthy life. Do your research and find a well-trained doctor in your area who can help you focus on *wellness* rather than *illness*.

Web Sites That Support Weight Loss

In today's world of instant information, sometimes all you need to know is which Web site to click on to support your journey to a healthier lifestyle. Here are a few of my favorites.

Before dining out, go to http://healthydiningfinder.com. If you know the name of the restaurant you would like patronize, just click on a letter at the top to see if it is included in this guide. Small local restaurants may not be listed.

I like to know the number of calories I will burn when I ride my bike for one hour at 11 miles per hour. Check this site to find that and much more: http://caloriescount.com/free_getmoving.aspx; all you have to do is input the activity, the time you will spend, and your age. Push the button and up comes the approximate number of calories you will burn. Note from the site: Figures are based on moderate (as opposed to vigorous) activity. A heavier person burns more calories, so the same amount of physical activity can actually burn the same number of calories, but more quickly. However, remember that exercising harder and faster only increases the calories expended slightly. To burn more calories, it is better to exercise for a longer time. Determining how many calories you burn is not an exact science. This number should only be used as an estimate of caloric expenditure.

Every five years the USDA puts out a food guide that sets food policy and educates the public on the latest nutritional research. Health professionals use this as a key guideline for their recommendations. Here is the USDA's most recent update: http://www.cnpp.usda.gov/Publications/DietaryGuidelines/2010/PolicyDoc/PolicyDoc.pdf.

It's all the small steps that have helped me weave my way though the challenges of a society filled with calorie-laden food. Learning what my body needs and when it needs it is critical to keeping it fueled so I don't consume more calories than I need. I am always on the lookout for a new idea that will support me in my new eating habits. The more I practice these steps that have helped me succeed, the more they become my way of life.

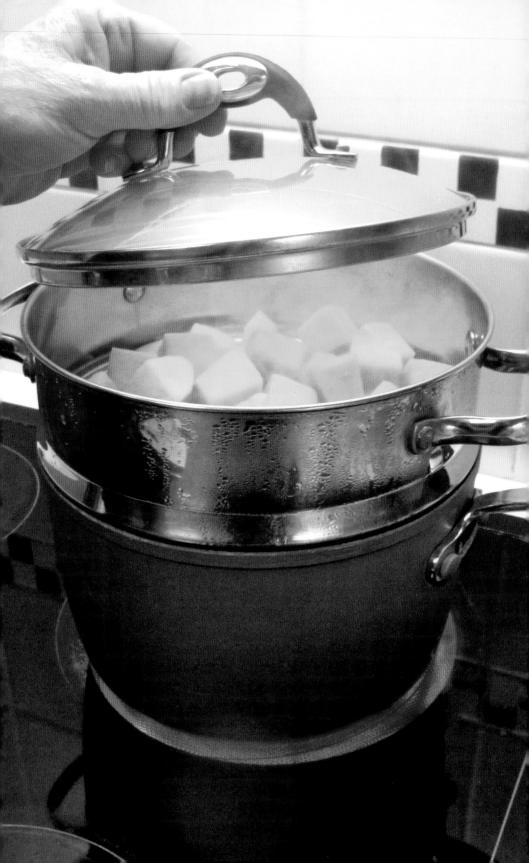

Chapter 6
Cooking Techniques & Ingredients

Healthy cooking doesn't mean you have to become a gourmet chef. Your choice of cooking techniques can reduce fat and calories. Consider that each tablespoon of butter or oil you use when frying adds 14 grams of fat and more than 100 calories. Even "light" olive oil derives 100 percent of its calories from fat.

Here are some methods that capture the flavor and retain the nutrients in your food without adding excessive amounts of fat or salt:

Braising: This involves browning the meat, poultry, or fish first, then adding a liquid, such as water or broth, covering the pan, and cooking it over low heat until it's tenderized. The cooking liquid usually becomes a flavorful sauce. Some examples are Chicken Cacciatore or beef pot roast. Slow cookers (also known as Crock-Pots) are a form of braising because the cooking liquid is retained in the food, keeping it moist.

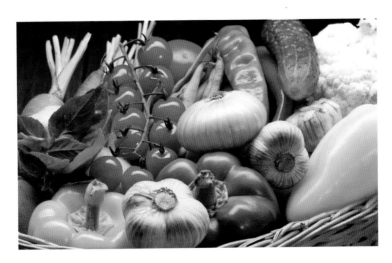

Grilling and Broiling: Both grilling and broiling expose food to direct, high heat. To grill outdoors, place the food on a rack above a bed of charcoal embers or gas flame. Avoid allowing the outside of the meat to char, or to be exposed to high heat for any extended period of time. You may want to start your grilling on foil, and then transfer the item to the grill for last-minute grill marks. For smaller items such as chopped vegetables, use foil or a long-handled grill basket to prevent pieces from slipping through the rack. To broil indoors, place food on a broiler rack below a heat element. Both methods allow fat to drip away from the food. The George Foreman Grill is an example of an indoor, electric contact grill that helps minimize the fat that stays in the meat.

Microwaving: This can be a quick, easy way to cook, especially if you are preparing a single serving. Microwaves can cook un-evenly, however. Arrange food items evenly in a microwaveable dish and add a small amount of liquid, if needed. Cover the dish and vent it. The moist heat created will help destroy harmful bacteria and help the item cook more uniformly. Stir or rotate food midway through the microwaving time to eliminate cold spots. Cooking times will vary with your oven's power and efficiency. Allow "standing time," where the food sits for a few minutes just after cooking. Be sure to use only cookware and plastic wrap that are considered safe for the microwave.

Boiling or Poaching: Both techniques involve cooking in water or other liquid. With boiling, the water comes to a boil, such as when you're cooking pasta. To poach foods, gently simmer ingredients in water or a flavorful liquid such as broth, vinegar, or juice until they're cooked through and tender. For stove-top poaching, choose a covered pan that best fits the size and shape of the food so that you need a minimal amount of liquid.

Roasting: Like baking, roasting uses an oven's dry heat to cook the food. You can roast foods on a baking sheet, in a roasting pan, or even outdoors in a Dutch oven. For poultry, seafood, and meat, place a rack inside the roasting pan so that the fat in the food can drip off during cooking. In some cases, you may need to baste it to keep it from drying out. For vegetables, toss them with a little olive oil, place on a baking sheet at around 400° F, and stir occasionally until the vegetables are tender and slightly browned. At any housewares store you can buy an oil spritzer that sprays a fine mist of pure oil over the vegetables, cutting down on the amount of oil needed.

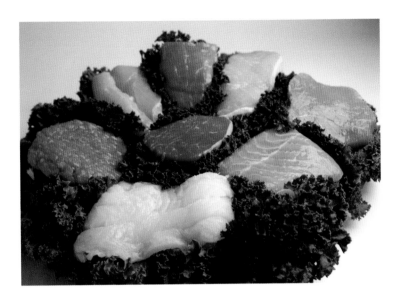

Sautéing: Sautéing cooks relatively small or thin pieces of food quickly. You can cook food using little or no oil. Depending on the recipe, use low-sodium broth, cooking spray, or water in place of oil.

Steaming: Place the food in a perforated basket suspended above simmering liquid. If you use a flavorful liquid or add seasonings to the water, you'll flavor the food as it cooks. You can use a double boiler with a steaming basket or an electric steamer.

Stir-frying: A traditional Asian method, stir-frying quickly cooks small, uniform-sized pieces of food over high heat while they are being stirred rapidly in a wok. You need only a small amount of oil or cooking spray for this method.

Whatever method you use, foods should be cooked to the following safe minimum internal temperatures:

Beef, veal, and lamb steaks and chops: 140° F for rare, 160° F for well done. Never serve meats that have an internal temperature of less than 140° F.
All cuts of pork: 145° F for medium, 160° F for well done.
Ground beef, veal, and lamb to 160° F.
Egg dishes, casseroles to 160° F.
Leftovers to 165° F.
Chicken, turkey, and other poultry to 165° F.

Super Seasonings

Spices and herbs add flavor and zest to foods so you can cut back on salt, fat, or sugar. There's also emerging evidence that with each pinch, dash, and spoonful, spices and herbs can help boost the antioxidant power of your food. Some studies suggest spices and herbs may help curb your hunger and stoke your metabolism as well.

Antioxidants boost our immune system and appear to reduce inflammation. Antioxidants are measured by ORAC, or oxygen radical absorbance capacity. Below is a list of some top seasonings for ORAC capacity, health properties, and flavor appeal.

You can buy many herbs and spices already combined, such as Italian seasoning, curry powder, Greek seasoning, and spice rubs. But be aware that some of them can be high in salt. Check the ingredients label; if salt is the first ingredient listed, this seasoning is high in sodium.

Most of the time, you just want a hint of flavor. If you add too much seasoning, you can end up with food that's bitter, pungent, or too hot. Mix in a pinch or two of the herb or spice, wait a few minutes for the flavors to blend, and then taste. It's easier to add a little more flavor than to remove it.

Cinnamon: One teaspoon of cinnamon contains as many antioxidants as a half-cup of blueberries, according to the spice company McCormick. Sprinkle ground cinnamon on your morning oatmeal, or on apple, peach, or pear slices. Toast whole-wheat bread, spread it with cottage cheese, and top it with a dash of cinnamon.

Black pepper: It's the most commonly used spice worldwide, and its extracts have been used as a folk medicine in many cultures. Some research links black pepper to enhancing digestive tract function. There's also some evidence that black pepper contains antioxidant, anti-inflammatory, and antimicrobial properties.

A hint of pepper perks up just about everything from vegetables to pasta to salad. Some folks love it sprinkled on strawberries, with a little brown sugar and balsamic vinegar.

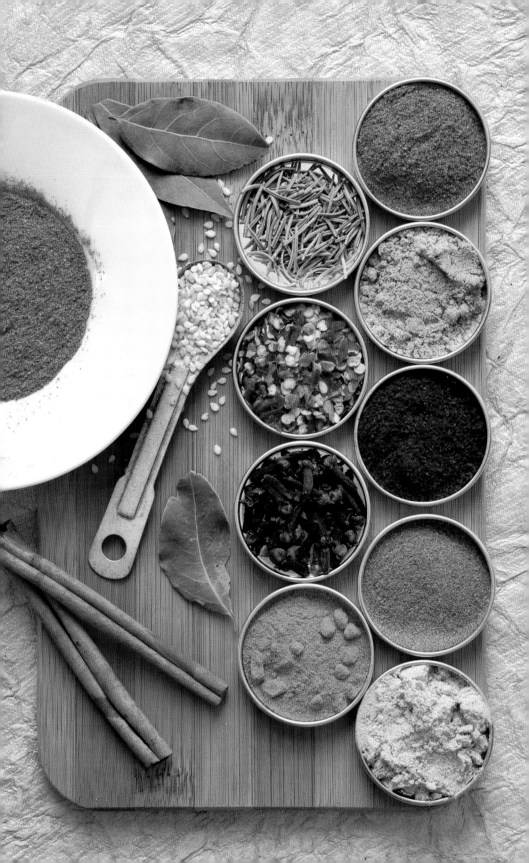

Turmeric: This bright gold spice is a cornerstone of curry powder. A teaspoon of curry powder has as many antioxidants as a half-cup of red grapes, according to McCormick.

Curcumin, the bright yellow compound in turmeric, has been shown to exhibit antioxidant, anti-inflammatory, antiviral, antibacterial, antifungal, and anticancer activities.

Mix ½ teaspoon of curry powder in 8 ounces of plain nonfat yogurt to spread on turkey and vegetable pita sandwiches. Add ½ teaspoon of curry powder to 2 cups of tomato soup. Stir a pinch into steamed brown rice, and top with toasted sliced almonds, shredded carrots, peas, and/or raisins. Lightly dust air-popped popcorn with curry powder.

Oregano: A Mediterranean mainstay, oregano has one of the highest antioxidant levels of all dried herbs. Just one teaspoon of dried oregano leaves has as many antioxidants as three ounces of almonds and one-half cup of chopped asparagus.

Sprinkle sautéed cherry or grape tomatoes with oregano, garlic powder, and salt and pepper to taste. Use a little with ground turkey to make Greek turkey burgers. It's also tasty sprinkled on fish, chicken, and pork.

Cumin: The flavor of this earthy spice plays a major role in Mexican, Thai, Vietnamese, and Indian cuisines. It is a critical ingredient of chili powder and is also found in curry powder, garam masala, and adobo seasonings.

Cumin adds flavor to low-fat dips such as hummus, black-bean dip, or salsa. Use it in spice rubs to flavor meats before grilling. Mix 1 tablespoon chili powder, 1½ teaspoons each of ground cumin, garlic powder, and oregano leaves, ¾ teaspoon of sea salt, and ¼ teaspoon each of ground black pepper and ground cinnamon. Rub onto pork tenderloins. Grill or roast until desired doneness.

Red chili pepper: Some studies have shown that when people added red pepper to their food, they ate fewer calories during that meal—and even during the next one. It is thought that capsaicin, the compound that gives chilies their heat, helps increase a feeling of fullness. Some studies indicate that spicing up your meal with cayenne, chili powder, and paprika can help boost your metabolism as well.

Add red chili powder to anything that needs a little kick. Be careful to add just a little, then taste before adding more. Unless you're a fan of fiery foods, you won't want to overdo it on the heat level.

Mix up your own spiced salt by combining 2 tablespoons of sea salt, 2 teaspoons of paprika, ½ teaspoon of ground cumin, and a pinch of ground red pepper. Sprinkle over grilled or roasted meat, fish, and poultry.

Ginger: This pungent, citrusy-flavored spice has as many antioxidants as a cup of spinach. For centuries, ginger was used as a natural remedy for a variety of conditions, especially soothing distressed stomachs. Now modern medicine is attempting to validate the use of ginger to ease indigestion and reduce pain.

Use a pinch of ground ginger in stir-frying, or try sprinkling it on peaches, pears, cantaloupe, pineapple, and honeydew melon.

Thyme: A teaspoon of this versatile herb contains about the same amount of antioxidants as a carrot or a half-cup of chopped tomatoes. Thyme also contains a variety of beneficial compounds called flavonoids. Throughout history, thyme was believed to have certain medicinal properties and was used to help treat chest and respiratory problems. A pinch of thyme adds a more complex flavor to soups, eggs, vegetables, meats, poultry, and seafood.

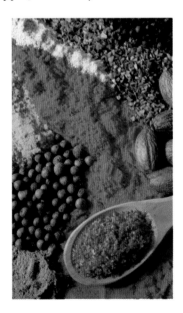

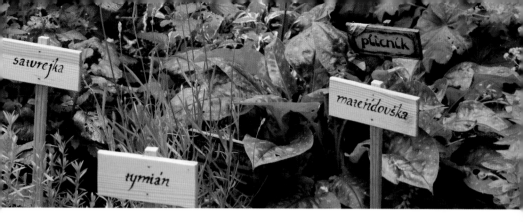

Rosemary: This classic Italian herb imparts a piney flavor. In ancient Greece, rosemary was thought to strengthen the brain and memory, and modern-day research has linked it to protection against brain degeneration.

Add ¼ teaspoon crushed rosemary leaves and ¼ teaspoon garlic to hot cooked peas or green beans. When you grill kebabs of chicken breast or lean meat cubes, thread them on sturdy sprigs of fresh rosemary. The sprigs infuse the meat from the inside out, and give a woodsy aroma while grilling as well.

Basil: This Italian herb is rich in carotenoids, a class of antioxidants. It also contains oils that prevent bacteria growth and inflammation.

Use basil in Italian dishes, eggs, and Italian soups such as minestrone. Make a lower-fat pesto by blending 2 cups of packed fresh basil leaves, 2 tablespoons of chopped almonds, 2 tablespoons of grated Parmesan, 2 tablespoons of olive oil, and 2 tablespoons of water. This is so flavorful that a little smear of it goes a long way in pasta, sandwiches, soups, and other Italian dishes.

Cilantro: This herb is a staple in Mexican, Thai, Middle Eastern, and South American cuisines. It has anti-inflammatory properties and is believed to aid digestion.

You'll want to use it fresh, as the dried version has very little flavor. Mix it into salsas, bean dips, and soups, or sprinkle some over meats to add both color and flavor.

Spice Blends: Spice blends are a convenient way to save you time and measuring. A brand I especially enjoy is NutriFit Salt & Sugar Free Spice Blends: Mediterranean, Lemon Garden, Certainly Cinnamon, Calypso, Rockin' Moroccan, and French Riviera. (See the following Web site: www.NutriFitonline.com.)

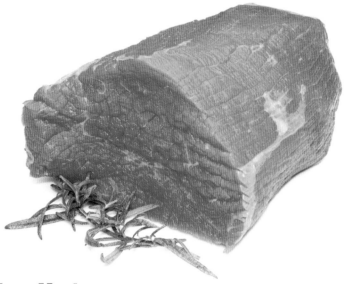

Lean Meats

When I adopted a healthier lifestyle, I began choosing leaner varieties and cuts of meat and measured portions.

White-meat poultry and many types of seafood are naturally lean when the skin is removed and they are cooked without added fat. Chicken and turkey breast are especially lean. Heavily marbled (thin streaks of fat within the muscle) beef and lamb are high in fat and calories. Pork today is usually quite lean, depending on the cut. Here are the types of meat and cuts I typically prepare:

1. **Fish:** halibut, salmon, haddock, cod

2. **Chicken:** white meat (or breast)

3. **Pork:** pork loin, pork chops, sirloin, boneless top loin roast, bone-in sirloin roast, pork tenderloin

4. **Beef:** extra-lean ground beef, round, chuck, sirloin, flank, well-trimmed tri-tip roast, tenderloin

5. **Turkey:** white meat (or breast). Ground dark turkey thighs also contain little fat.

As soon as I get home from the grocery store, I trim all visible fat from the meat, divide it into single-serving sizes using my scale to weigh it, and freeze. Family-size portions can be calculated by determining the appropriate serving size for each family member and adding up the total ounces.

At the beginning of the week I remove my frozen meats, place them in a plastic container in the fridge, and let them thaw. It is important to remove as much air as possible from freezer bags or containers when storing meat to prevent freezer burn. Frozen meat should be used within six months.

The following are calories (approximate) for three ounces cooked without added fat:

Chicken, skinless, white meat	138 calories
Turkey, skinless, white meat	132 calories
Haddock	95 calories
Halibut	119 calories
Tuna canned in water	99 calories
Crab, Alaska King	82 calories
Shrimp	121 calories
Salmon	129 calories
Beef, bottom round	178 calories
Beef, top round	157 calories
Beef, chuck blade pot roast	213 calories
Beef, top sirloin	165 calories
Beef, flank steak	220 calories
Beef, tenderloin	185 calories
Beef, ground, 85 percent lean	217 calories
Beef, ground, 90 percent lean	196 calories
Pork, tenderloin	133 calories
Pork chops, center loin or top loin chop	165 calories
Pork, boneless top loin	162 calories
Pork, bone-in sirloin roast	121 calories

OTHER PROTEIN

1 large egg	80 calories
1 large egg white	17 calories
Egg beaters (egg whites), ¼ cup	30 calories
Veggie burger patty, 2.5 ounces	70 to 170 calories, depending on the brand

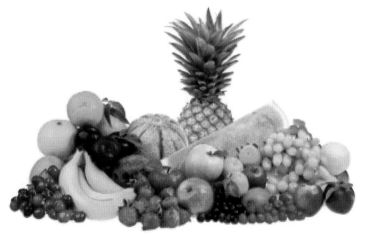

Fabulous Fruits

Ever since I started losing weight, I have been looking for delicious, nutritious ways to prepare fruits. When eating out, if I discover a fruit dish I like, I ask for the recipe. Most restaurants are happy to share them.

Fruits have many vital vitamins and nutrients, but you should try to follow the proper serving sizes. Some fruits have concentrated sugars and can add more calories than you think.

I eat citrus fruit—an orange, grapefruit, or Clementine—every day, as well as two other servings of fruit. Crushed berries make a delicious sauce to spoon over fat-free yogurt or nonfat cottage cheese.

Most fruits store well in the refrigerator for several days. Some fruits, such as bananas, are picked green and continue to ripen, so they should be set on the counter.

If I don't eat soft fruits, such as peaches and nectarines, within a few days, I peel them, cut them into 1-inch pieces, place them on a piece of plastic wrap on a tray, and freeze them uncovered. Then I divide the pieces into serving portions and package them in Ziploc freezer bags, removing as much air from the bags as possible before sealing. When frozen, they are ready to use in fruit shakes.

One serving equals ½ cup of fruit, 1 medium piece of fruit, ¼ cup of dried fruit, or 6 ounces of 100 percent fruit juice.

Apple, 1 medium	72 calories
Avocado, ¼ of one avocado	80 calories
Banana, 1 medium	90 calories
Blueberries, ½ cup	83 calories
Cantaloupe or honeydew, ½ cup	25 calories
Cherries, ½ cup	37 calories
Grapes, ½ cup	31 calories
Grapefruit, ½ large	60 calories
Kiwi, 1 medium	100 calories
Orange, 1 medium	60 calories
Peach, 1 medium	38 calories
Pineapple, ½ cup	39 calories
Plum, 1	30 calories
Prunes, dried, 3	60 calories
Raisins or other dried fruit, ¼ cup	108 calories
Strawberries, frozen, thawed, ½ cup	38 calories
Raspberries or boysenberries, ½ cup	32 calories
Watermelon, ½ cup, diced	46 calories

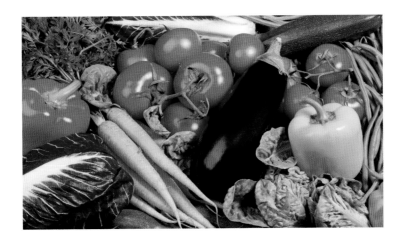

Valuable Vegetables

You will want to eat as many vegetables as you can. Most are low in calories and high in vitamins, minerals, antioxidants, and fiber. According to the USDA, the serving size for raw leafy greens is 1 cup; the serving size for other raw or cooked vegetables is ½ cup. So a generous-sized salad containing two cups of spring greens and another cup of chopped raw vegetables would give you three servings of vegetables.

Artichoke hearts, canned in water, ½ cup	45 calories
Artichokes, fresh, boiled, 1 medium	60 calories
Asparagus, fresh, cooked, ½ cup or 5 spears	20 calories
Avocado, ½ cup, cubed	120 calories
Beets, cooked, ½ cup	37 calories
Broccoli, ½ cup, chopped	30 calories
Brussels sprouts, ½ cup, cooked	28 calories
Carrots, ½ cup, raw strips	25 calories
Cauliflower, ½ cup, raw	13 calories
Celery, ½ cup, diced	8 calories
Corn, ½ cup, cooked, or 1 medium ear	66 calories
Cucumber, ½ cup, sliced, raw with peel	8 calories
Green beans, ½ cup, raw	22 calories
Kale, 1 cup, chopped	34 calories
Leeks, ½ cup, lower leaf portion	27 calories

Lettuce (iceberg), 1 cup, shredded	8 calories
Lettuce (romaine), 1 cup	10 calories
Mushrooms, ½ cup, raw pieces	15 calories
Olives, ½ cup, ripe, canned, black	80 calories
Onions, ½ cup, chopped	32 calories
Peas, ½ cup, raw	62 calories
Peppers, bell, 1 large	50 calories
Potato, baked, 1 medium	161 calories
Radishes, ½ cup, sliced	9 calories
Squash (winter), ½ cup, cubed	21 calories
Spinach, 1 cup, raw	7 calories
Sugar snap peas, ⅔ cup, raw	37 calories
Tomato, 1 small	19 calories
Tomato, ½ cup, chopped	38 calories
Yam or sweet potato, ½ cup	79 calories
Zucchini, ½ cup, chopped	10 calories
Vegetable juice, 6 ounces	35 calories

Whole Grains

Whole grains include the entire grain seed, usually called the kernel. The kernel consists of three components—the bran, germ, and endosperm. Whole grains are consumed either as a single food (such as wild rice or popcorn) or as an ingredient in foods (cereals, breads, and crackers). Some examples of whole-grain ingredients include buckwheat, bulgur, millet, oatmeal, quinoa, rolled oats, brown or wild rice, whole-grain barley, whole rye, and whole wheat.

Refined grains have been milled to remove the bran and germ from the grain. This is done to give grains a finer texture and improve their shelf life, but milling also removes dietary fiber, iron, and many B vitamins.

For your weight-loss program, choose products made with whole grains, including cereals, pasta, breads, and so on.

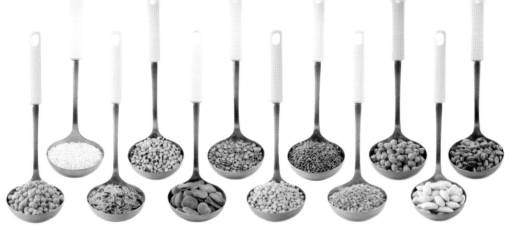

Whole-wheat bread, 1 slice	80 to 100 calories
Whole-wheat bagel, ½ (1 ounce)	135 calories
Whole-wheat roll, 1 small (1 ounce)	140 calories
Corn tortilla, 1 six-inch diameter	65 calories
Cold cereals, 1 ounce	80–250 calories, depending on the type
Whole-grain cereals (oatmeal, cracked wheat), ½ cup, cooked	120–150 calories
Brown rice, ½ cup, cooked	108 calories
Whole-wheat pasta or Soba noodles, ½ cup, cooked	88 calories
Popcorn, 1 cup, air-popped	31 calories
Pretzels, whole wheat, 1 ounce	101 calories

Beans and Legumes

Beans are the mature forms of legumes. They include kidney beans, pinto beans, black beans, garbanzo beans (chickpeas), lima beans, black-eyed peas, split peas, and lentils.

Beans are excellent sources of protein. They also provide other nutrients, such as iron and zinc, also found in seafood, meat, and poultry. They are excellent sources of dietary fiber and nutrients such as potassium and folate, which also are found in other vegetables. Because of their high nutrient content, beans may be considered both as a vegetable and as a protein food.

Black beans, ½ cup, cooked or canned	100 calories
Navy beans, ½ cup, cooked or canned	108 calories
Kidney beans, ½ cup, cooked	109 calories
Pinto beans, ½ cup, cooked	103 calories
Garbanzo beans, ½ cup, cooked	143 calories
Split peas, ½ cup, cooked	116 calories
Lentils, ½ cup, cooked	115 calories

Dairy

Dairy products contribute many nutrients for good health, such as calcium, vitamin D, and potassium, and are linked to strong bones. The 2010 Dietary Guidelines for Americans recommends three cups per day of fat-free or low-fat milk products.

Fat-free milk, yogurt, and cottage cheese provide the same nutrients with less fat and fewer calories.

Fat-free milk, 8 ounces (1 cup)	86 calories
Light or reduced-fat soy milk, 8 ounces (1 cup)	60 calories
Nonfat plain yogurt, 8 ounces (1 cup)	100 calories
Nonfat fruit-flavored yogurt, 8 ounces (1 cup)	213 calories
Nonfat cottage cheese, ½ cup	80 calories
Cheese, Cheddar, 1 ounce	114 calories
Cheese, part-skim mozzarella, 1 ounce	72 calories
Cheese, reduced fat, 1 ounce	80 calories
Grated Parmesan cheese, ¼ cup	110 calories

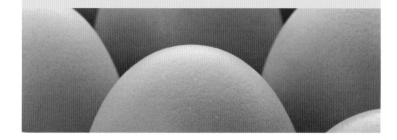

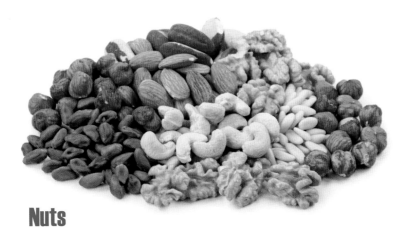

Nuts

Nuts are high in fat, but the oil is heart-healthy. Many studies, including one done at the Harvard School of Public Health, found that nuts may help lower cholesterol if they replace less healthy foods in the diet. Nuts contain mono- and polyunsaturated fats known to benefit the heart. They also contain fiber and vitamin E.

Nuts are high in calories, but the Harvard study theorized that just two ounces of nuts per week are all that are needed to help lower heart disease risk. Avoid nuts that are fried in oil or loaded with salt.

Peanuts, technically a legume (a dried pea, bean, or lentil), are usually included in the nut group because they have a similar nutrient profile. Typically, one ounce of nuts fits into the palm of your hand.

Nuts (shelled and roasted):	
Mixed, 1 ounce	170 calories
Almonds, 1 ounce, whole	163 calories
Peanuts, dry-roasted, 1 ounce	166 calories
Cashews, 1 ounce	156 calories
Walnuts, 1 ounce	185 calories
Pistachio nuts, 1 ounce	161 calories
Sunflower seeds, 1 ounce	165 calories
Pine nuts, 1 ounce	190 calories
Reduced-fat peanut butter, 1 tablespoon	83 calories
Peanut butter, creamy, 1 tablespoon	105 calories
Peanut butter, super chunk, 1 tablespoon	90 calories
Soy nuts, ⅓ cup	140 calories

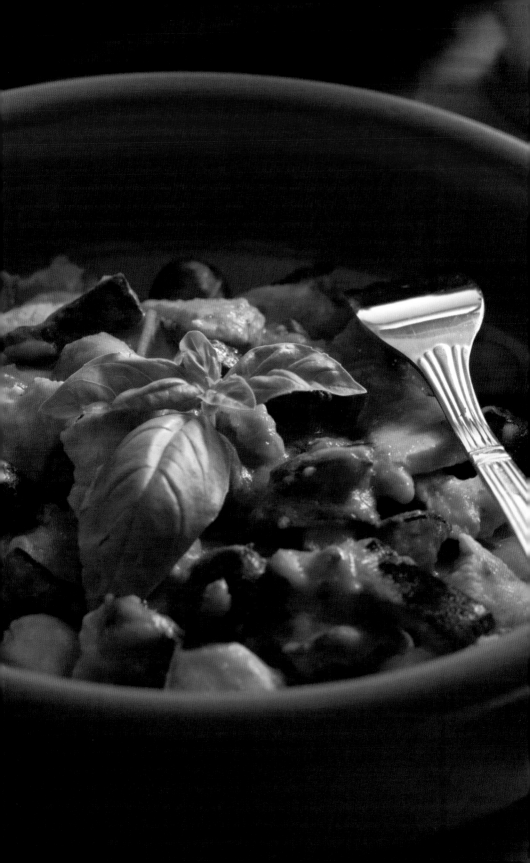

Chapter 7
Meal Planning Keys to Successful Weight Loss

Planning meals and snacks in advance will set you up for success. Through the years, and with much practice, this routine has become easier for me. Plan what you will eat for the whole week.

A woman called me the other day and began our conversation with "I weigh 320 pounds. That is in the range of what you weighed when you started your weight-loss program." She went on to tell me she had lost 90 pounds once, then gained it back, and lost 50 again, which also came right back. This story could be told over and over, as people look for diets and quick fixes.

A diet can be compared to holding a glass of water in the air. You can hold it up for only so long—sooner or later you'll have to put it down. Yes, a lucky few keep the weight off, but the percentages are low. You can check the statistics online at The National Weight Control Registry, which has tracked the weight loss and weight maintenance of over 2,600 people all across the country. To me, losing weight is also like taking piano lessons. It starts with incorporating small, simple steps, and then requires consistent practicing before the weight comes off and stays off.

When I was eating without considering the consequences, just about any tempting-looking food crossed my lips. Jackie gave me tasks each week to practice and master. Making consistent progress took time and energy to implement what I was learning. The many small steps I took literally made a new me. Many of the contestants on the popular television show *The Biggest Loser* regain the weight when they leave the ranch. Losing weight slowly allows your body to accommodate the many changes that

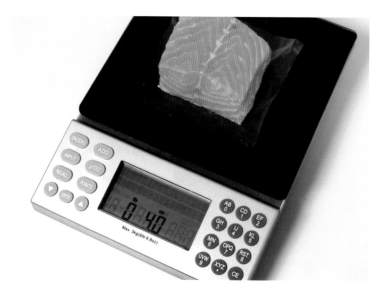

will take place. A plastic surgeon once told me I shouldn't lose more than a pound a week because the body needs time to adjust the joints, bones, and skin.

One of the main keys for me is setting up the food in advance so I can come into the kitchen and prepare a healthy meal in 15 minutes or less. This takes careful planning, shopping, and then prepping the food for the week. I often use the kitchen scales to help me weigh out my portions. I find eating the right things in the proper portions is the most important step. This chapter contains sample menus that will give you an idea of the types of foods and the amounts you can eat to lose weight.

How many calories do I need? At 5' 8" with a medium to large frame, I should eat between 1,700 and 1,800 calories to lose weight. Eating nutritionally dense food prevents me from getting really hungry. Your first step will be to determine how many calories you should eat and how much exercise you will need to lose weight. The Surgeon General recommends that people get at least 150 minutes of moderate to intense exercise per week—30 minutes per day for at least five days per week. In 2011, this 2009 recommendation was updated, with the change of adding strength training to your fitness routine at least two days per week. Health coaches, dietitians, exercise experts, and medical specialists can assist in refining these numbers to match your needs. Be sure to check with your physician before making any extreme changes in diet and exercise.

There are also many Internet sites that can give you guidance. For example, http://www.mypyramid.gov/ provides the recommended USDA guideline for you. It also gives ideas for each category of recommendations.

While losing weight I've been consistently performing strength-training and cardiovascular exercises. This has helped my endurance and muscle mass increase, which in turn helps me to burn more calories during my daily activities and while resting.

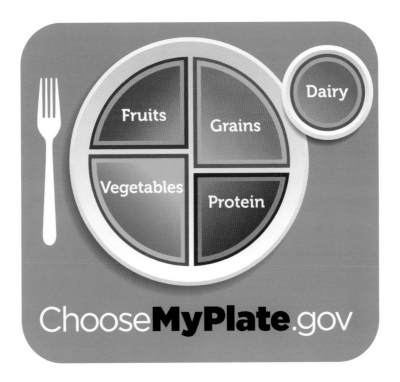

Breaking the Fast

Many Americans do not eat breakfast, even though nutritionists say that breakfast is the most important meal of the day. You've probably heard the old adage: Eat like a king at breakfast, a prince at lunch, and a pauper at dinner.

Unless you're Dagwood Bumstead, your body has been without food for more than eight hours. The very definition of breakfast is "breaking the fast."

Eating a good breakfast gives your body the fuel it needs to get off to an optimal start. Those who choose to skip breakfast may have an energy drop and are more inclined to overeat the wrong foods later.

My breakfast goal is to avoid later-in-the-day binge eating by consuming a fat, a complex carbohydrate, and some protein each morning. And I strive to hold this meal to about 350 calories.

Here are some of my typical breakfasts:

Breakfast 1

1 scrambled egg cooked without added butter or salt. Instead use cooking spray.

1 slice whole-wheat toast, dry, or with ½ teaspoon of trans-fat-free, light spread (such as Smart Balance Light), or 1 tablespoon high-quality, sugar-free jam (such as Cornaby's 10-Calorie Spreadable Fruit).

½ cup salsa. Homemade is best, as you can minimize the salt. Regular salsa has about 780 mg sodium/serving. If using commercially prepared salsa, make sure there's less than 140 mg sodium/serving.

1 fruit. Any seasonal fruit will work, or substitute ½ cup of canned (in juice, not syrup) fruit of your choice.

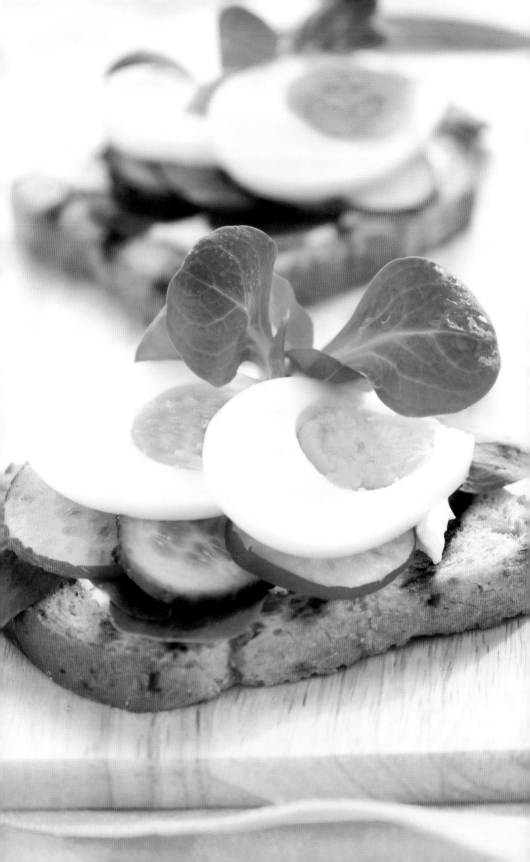

Breakfast 2

1 cup fat-free cottage cheese, or one cup plain, fat-free yogurt (regular or Greek, no sugar added).

1 slice whole-wheat toast, dry, or with ½ teaspoon of trans-fat-free, light spread (such as Smart Balance Light), or 1 tablespoon high-quality, sugar-free jam (such as Cornaby's 10-Calorie Spreadable Fruit).

1 fruit. Any seasonal fruit will work, or substitute ½ cup of canned (in juice, not syrup) fruit of your choice.

Breakfast 3

1 tablespoon fat-free cream cheese.

2 ounces smoked salmon. Always check the sodium content in smoked fish! Try to find one with less than 300 mg sodium/serving.

1 slice whole-wheat toast, dry, or with ½ teaspoon of trans-fat-free, light spread (such as Smart Balance Light), or 1 tablespoon high-quality, sugar-free jam (such as Cornaby's 10-Calorie Spreadable Fruit).

1 fruit. Any seasonal fruit will work, or substitute ½ cup of canned (in juice, not syrup) fruit of your choice.

Breakfast 4

1 cup fat-free plain yogurt, or 1 cup fat-free Greek yogurt (unsweetened). If you prefer fruit-flavored yogurt, use a type of yogurt that is fruit-juice sweetened, rather than sweetened with high-fructose corn syrup or sugar.

1 slice whole-wheat toast, dry, or with ½ teaspoon of trans-fat-free, light spread (such as Smart Balance Light), or 1 tablespoon high-quality, sugar-free jam (such as Cornaby's 10-Calorie Spreadable Fruit).

1 tablespoon reduced-fat peanut butter. Select a brand that has less than 11–12 g fat per serving.

1 fruit. Any seasonal fruit will work, or substitute ½ cup of canned (in juice, not syrup) fruit of your choice.

Breakfast 5

½ cup Grape-Nuts.
1 cup skim milk.
1 apple.

Breakfast 6

1 cup oatmeal (or other whole-grain cereal), cooked, without butter or sugar.

1 cup fat-free milk. You can prepare the oatmeal with milk instead of water, if desired.

1 fruit. Any seasonal fruit will work, or substitute ½ cup of canned (in juice, not syrup) fruit of your choice.

Breakfast 7

2 (4-inch) whole-wheat pancakes (about 170 calories with 3 g fat and 5 g fiber), no butter or syrup.

1 egg, scrambled, without added butter or salt. Instead, use cooking spray, extra-virgin olive oil spray, or canola oil spray and add fresh herbs or a salt-free seasoning blend.

½ cup pineapple. Select fresh or canned pineapple in 100 percent fruit juice, not canned in syrup.

½ banana.

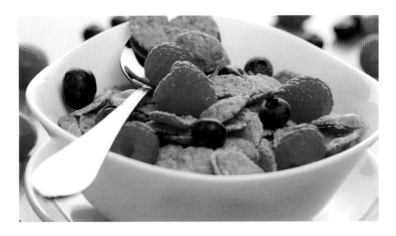

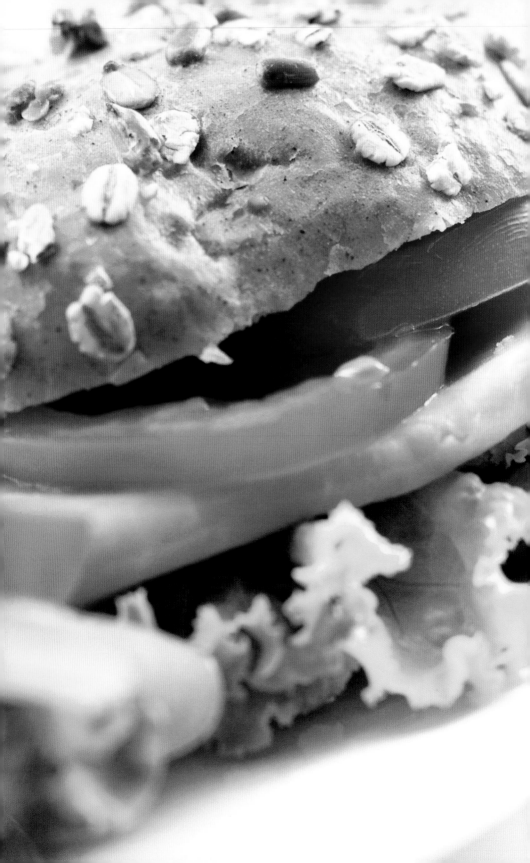

Power Lunches

Lunch is a vital key in keeping your energy up throughout the day. If you have lunch away from home, it's wise to plan and prepare ahead of time. If lunch is not well-thought-out in advance, you may get distracted and not eat at all, or eat the wrong foods. A friend of mine works at various locations all the time. She plans and prepares healthy lunches to pack in her cooler every day. Remember, if you fail to eat, you set yourself up for an energy drop in the afternoon and an all-blowout meal at dinner.

Here is a sampling of my lunch menus.

Lunch 1

3 ounces salmon canned in water, drained well.
1 tablespoon nonfat Miracle Whip (juice of lemon can also be used).
1 slice whole-wheat bread.
2 medium carrots.
1 rib celery.
½ roasted pepper (roasted on the grill or in the oven). If you prefer, substitute another celery rib.
Lettuce or spinach to go on bread slice.

Lunch 2

3 ounces cooked chicken breast.
3 cups spring greens.
2 tablespoons lite dressing.
1 cup steamed vegetables.
1 slice whole-wheat toast, dry, or with ½ teaspoon of trans-fat-free, light spread (such as Smart Balance Light).

Lunch 3

4 ounces raw extra-lean ground beef or turkey (cooked and seasoned with a spice blend and without salt).
1 whole-wheat bun (choose one with approximately 100 calories).
Leaves of lettuce or spinach to go on burger (as much as you like).
2 slices tomato.
1 slice sweet onion (optional).
Raw vegetables (2 medium carrots, or as much celery, cucumber, or pepper as you like).

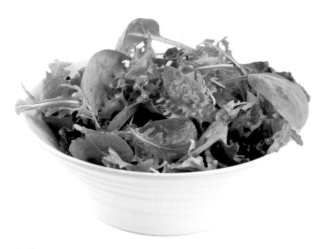

Lunch 4

2 cups hearty Mexican Soup (see recipe on page 169).
1 tablespoon hard cheese.
2 6-inch corn tortillas (40 to 50 calories each).

Lunch 5

2 hard-cooked eggs (made into an egg salad).
1 tablespoon nonfat Miracle Whip.
1 teaspoon mustard (optional).
1 slice whole-wheat toast, dry, or with ½ teaspoon of trans-fat-free, light
   spread (such as Smart Balance Light).
Mixed green salad with lite dressing.

Lunch 6

1½ cups homemade chili with vegetables. You might want to stir up a
   big pot of this and freeze it in single-serving packages.
1 slice whole-wheat bread or toast, dry, or with ½ teaspoon of trans-
   fat-free, light spread (such as Smart Balance Light).
1 piece fruit.

Lunch 7

2 cups vegetable soup.
1 slice whole-wheat bread or toast, dry, or with ½ teaspoon of trans-fat-
   free light spread (such as Smart Balance Light).

Delicious Dinners

Dinner is generally the meal most people have time to prepare and enjoy, a wonderful opportunity to have the family sit down and eat together. When cooking for myself I often prepare extra for tasty leftovers. I have learned that when I prepare foods for future meals, it is a good idea to portion them out and put them directly into the refrigerator so I'm not overeating at dinner. It is also wise to turn off the TV so that you can concentrate on your meal.

Here are some of the dinners that I enjoy. I usually start with 4 oz. of raw meat (3 oz. cooked) with two to three vegetables and a small green salad if I haven't eaten one during the day. If you love salad, have it twice a day—the more vegetables you eat, the better!

Dinner 1

4 ounces salmon.
Spring greens salad with bell pepper, shredded carrot, and sliced mushrooms.
1 cup butternut squash, steamed.
3 cups raw baby spinach (will become about 1 cup steamed).

Dinner 2

4 ounces extra-lean ground beef or turkey, pan-fried.
½ cup whole-wheat pasta, cooked.
1 cup seasoned tomato sauce.
1 cup asparagus, steamed.
2 tablespoons grated Parmesan cheese.
2 tablespoons lite dressing.

Dinner 3

4 ounces pork loin chop, grilled on barbecue or pan-fried.
½ potato or sweet potato, microwaved or steamed.
1 roasted pepper, grilled on barbecue or broiled.
Green salad.
2 tablespoons lite dressing.

Dinner 4

Stir-fry made from:
4 ounces lean pork, beef, or chicken.
3 to 4 vegetables for stir-fry (see chart on page 181).
2 tablespoons Newman's Own Lighten Up Low Fat Sesame Ginger Dressing (sauce for stir-fry).

Dinner 5

4 ounces pork loin, cubed and pan-fried; then remove from stove and add after onion and cabbage are cooked (see recipe on page 185).
1 medium onion, caramelized.
3 cups shredded red cabbage, raw (stirred in with onions after they are caramelized).
2 tablespoons prepared mustard.

Dinner 6

4 ounces white fish, pan-fried.
$^3/_4$ cup Brussels sprouts, steamed.
1 sweet pepper, grilled on barbecue or broiled.
1 cup acorn squash, steamed.

Dinner 7

4 ounces lean steak, pan-fried and seasoned to taste.
1 cup broccoli, steamed.
Spring greens salad with grated carrot, diced celery, and sliced mushrooms (or whatever vegetables you have on hand).
1 cup squash, steamed.

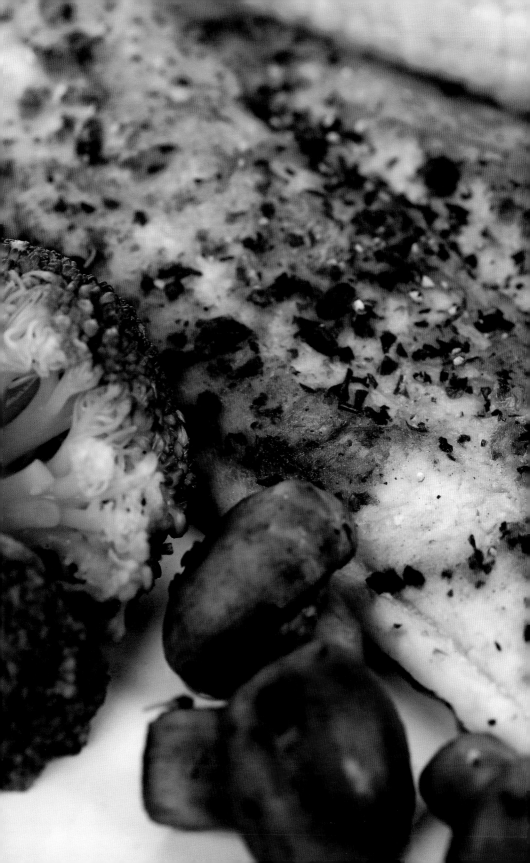

Snacks That Satisfy

When I first started the program, Jackie taught me to eat three meals and three snacks each day. This made it much easier to last between eating times. It seems as though I have a good, healthy meal and before long, it's time for a snack.

A recent houseguest once said, "You really enjoy what you eat!" She's right. By planning nutritious and delicious meals and snacks ahead of time, I can sit back and enjoy my food in the healthy body that has resulted from making good food choices.

Healthy snacks should contain 150 calories. They give your body the energy it needs so you don't get too hungry and reach for the wrong foods, or overeat at the next meal.

Breakfast is between 7 a.m. and 8:30 a.m., lunch is between noon and 1:30 p.m., and dinner is between 5:30 and 7 p.m., with snacks halfway between each meal and the final one between 8 and 9 p.m.

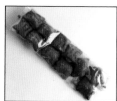
11 peanut butter pretzels

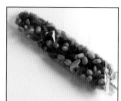
1 tablespoon each of dried fruit, soy nuts, pumpkin seeds, dark chocolate chips

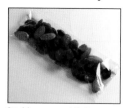
2 tablespoons dried cranberries or raisins and 10 almonds

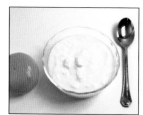
1 cup nonfat, sugar-free yogurt and 1 Clementine

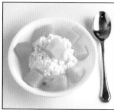
Half-cup nonfat cottage cheese and half-cup pineapple chunks

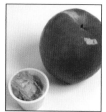
1 apple and 1 table-spoon reduced-fat peanut butter

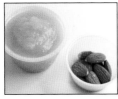

Half-cup applesauce and 10 almonds

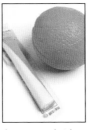

1 orange and string cheese

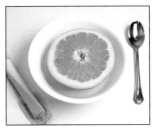

One-half grapefruit and string cheese

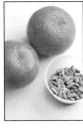

2 Clementines and two tablespoons sunflower seeds

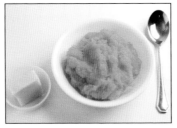

1 cup squash and one-half ounce cheese

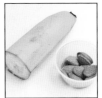

One-half banana and 10 almonds

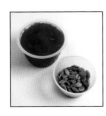

Half-cup blueberry-pomegranate applesauce and 2 tablespoons pumpkin seeds

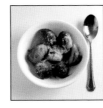

1 cup Brussels sprouts and 1 tablespoon grated hard cheese

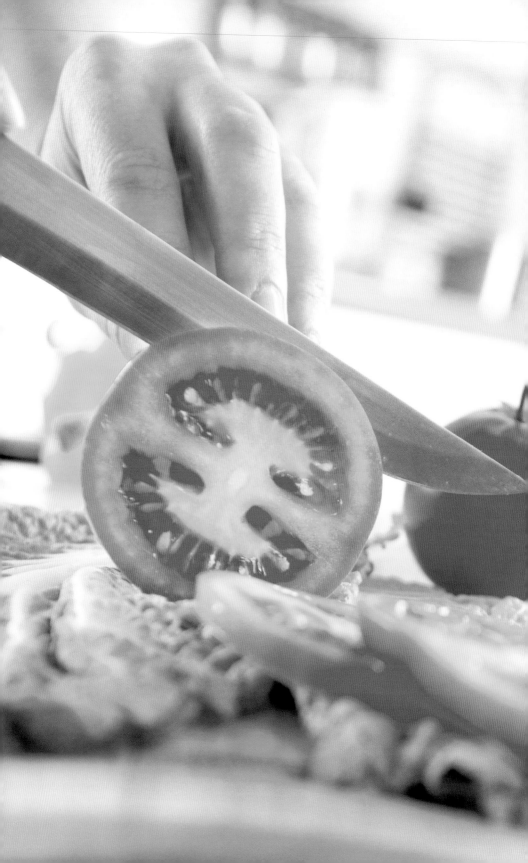

Chapter 8
Recipes

I seldom use recipes exactly as shown in the cookbook. I enjoy reading recipes for ideas, but I often find I don't have all the ingredients on hand, so following the recipe as written would require a trip to the store. On the few occasions I have shopped for those special or one-time-used ingredients, they have usually ended up wasting away in my refrigerator or cupboard for months until I eventually toss them out. To avoid that waste of time and money, I follow a recipe generally and make liberal substitutions.

On those rare occasions that I do need to follow a specific recipe, I conduct an Internet search and review all the ones that come up. I sometimes use the recipe as is, or I will construct my own. Key is finding the combinations of the ingredients that you enjoy.

Since beginning my new lifestyle, I prepare most of my meals at home, mainly from items found in the produce section. I take advantage of my supermarket's weekly bargains and design many of my meals around them. After returning home with my purchases, I prep the food for the week before refrigerating it. I like to have my food organized and ready for an entire week.

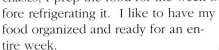

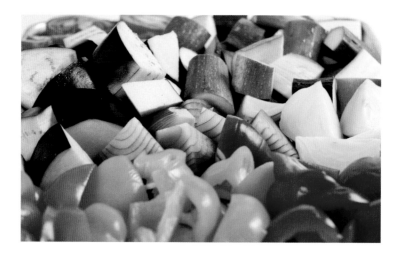

For example, I recently drove from St. George, Utah, to Salt Lake City. Mountainview Mushroom Farm is just off the freeway in Fillmore, about 90 miles south of Salt Lake. I decided to stop. Since they don't sell these delightfully fresh mushrooms in small quantities, I had to purchase a minimum of ten pounds. No problem, because I love mushrooms, especially these, which are harvested every morning. They are so fresh that the texture is much like an apple's. When they are that appealing, you don't mind having them for four or five meals. It was a bonus to have some to share.

In this section you will find some recipes that are written in the traditional manner, but I have also included charts and some basic directions for preparing stir-fry, soups, sandwiches, and salads that give you the freedom to use what you have on hand and what you like best. These four items are what I eat most of the time.

I invite you to become an artist with fresh vegetables and fruits. Remember back when you were a child with a new box of Crayons? It was fun and exciting to mix the new colors. This freedom to create new and innovative combinations, just like I did as a kid, has helped me immensely. Now I have many favorite "recipes" tailored just for me.

Since you can eat all the nonstarchy vegetables you want, try out a few flavor combinations and see what you come up with. For example, soon after returning home from Fillmore, I had a huge bowl of fresh sautéed mushrooms and onions topped with roasted tomato sauce sprinkled with a little grated hard cheese. What will you make?

Adding Flavor to Food

This past Christmas as I was listening to the list of gifts my nephew had received, one stood out. I went right to the computer and ordered *The Flavor Bible*. This incredible book was written by a husband and wife, Karen Page, a journalist, and Andrew Dornenburg, a chef.

As big as a Bible, it is a key reference for anyone who is looking for flavorful, unique combinations. Eight years in the making, *The Flavor Bible* is a landmark book that is sure to inspire cooking innovation. Cuisine is undergoing a startling historic transformation: with the advent of the global availability of ingredients, dishes are no longer based on geography but on flavor. Created by some of the best culinary artists in the American food world, *The Flavor Bible* is a guide to hundreds of ingredients plus herbs, spices, and other seasonings that will allow you to coax the greatest possible flavor and pleasure from them. If you have a creative flair, you will not want to be without this book. This is what I consulted after my mushroom purchase.

The book lists ingredients alphabetically. Under "M" I found mushroom. It then lists other ingredients, spices, and herbs that complement mushrooms. Ingredients that are highly recommended are in bold. When asparagus came up under "A," I said, "This is it!" I made a mouth-watering stir-fry using onions, asparagus, mushrooms, and precooked chicken. After adding a little tomato sauce and sprinkling on some grated hard cheese, I was set for a delicious, nutritious, low-calorie dish.

Throughout the book are delectable combinations that chefs and cooking experts have written about. These will give you more ideas to try than you could ever put together yourself. Check this out, written by Michael Laiskonis, owner of Le Bernardin in New York City: "Ginger is great on its own, but also works great with other flavors. It's one of those 'wake up' flavors that you can hide beneath all sorts of other flavors. I think it works especially well with citrus. It works with passion fruit, coconut, banana, and other tropical flavors." The book also lists flavor affinities, for example, ginger + carrot + celery + garlic.

If you like experimenting with foods and flavors, check *The Flavor Bible* out of your library, or ask for it next Christmas.

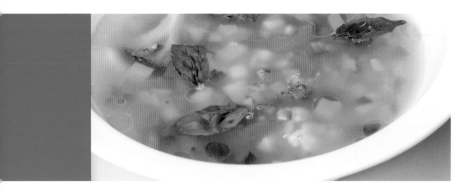

Soups and Stews

Soup is comfort food at its best. These one-pot wonders can be hot and spicy, chunky with meat and vegetables, or velvety smooth. Soups make it easy to work in a lot of different vegetables that you might not try on their own. Soups are also budget-friendly. A handful of ingredients can stretch to feed a crowd, and all those odds and ends left in the refrigerator can be tossed in to add color and flavor. Another benefit is that it will clean out your refrigerator of those vegetables you weren't sure where to use.

Soup-Making Tips

Guida Ponte shared with me some wonderful soup recipes and tips for making them. I met her when I was working on the *Today* show, and she was executive chef for the Legal Seafood restaurant, a popular chain in Boston. Hailing from the Azores, a group of Portuguese islands in the mid-Atlantic, she is a fabulous cook; if you can grow it, Guida can cook it. Today, her main job at Verrill Farm outside Boston is to make soups every day, which she has done for the past ten years. I asked her to share some of her best soup tips:

- If you are going to blend the soup, don't chop the garlic.
- Put the pan on the hot burner and let it heat up before adding any oil. That way it won't burn.
- If you don't want to use broth or stock, you can use water and add more seasoning to your soup.
- When boiling beans, you can add pepper, thyme, a bay leaf, garlic, or onions to give them extra flavor.

- Brown just about everything on high heat.
- When pureeing a soup in the blender, let it cool a little before blending.
- Slice veggies on the diagonal for an interesting appearance.
- Never add salt until the very end.
- Kosher salt has a better flavor than iodized salt.

Eat Pureed, Not Creamed, Soups

You can find a lot of calories in creamed soups; calories are added through butter, cream, and cheese. I have replaced all of my creamed soups with pureed soups made with a broth and vegetables. You can prepare your own broth, purchase canned or boxed stock, or use bouillon. Just be sure to watch the sodium content. When purchasing canned items, buy low-sodium types.

Once you master the technique for pureed soups, endless varieties can be made. Whether you add asparagus, squash, or any other vegetable, the procedure is similar. Your variables will include the spices you choose to add.

Gather Your Tools

1. A good pot
Don't underestimate the importance of a good, heavy pot. It's the most important equipment needed for making great soup. A heavy-bottomed pan will enable you to maintain a steady simmer and gentle boil without scorching.

2. A blender
A blender is important in making pureed soups. Blend the soup in batches, letting the blender run on a low speed for two to three minutes per batch. Use care as hot steam can sometimes build up and blow the blender lid off. Start on a slow speed, keeping the lid slightly ajar to vent steam. When the steam is vented, seal the lid and increase your blending speed. Place a small kitchen towel over the lid just in case there are splatters created from the heat pressure in the blender. In my opinion, the best blenders on the market are VitaMix® and Blendtec®.

3. A ladle
A long-handled ladle beats dishing soup out with a cup anytime.

MAKING PUREED SOUPS

1. Heat canola oil (no more than a tablespoon) in soup pot over medium heat.
2. Add aromatics (onions, leeks, and/or garlic) with your key fresh vegetables to warmed canola oil and cover. This process is called "sweating" the vegetables. The vegetables are ready when they are soft, give off a little steam, and are brightly colored. Onions should be translucent and golden, not brown. This should only take a few minutes, so don't wander off to watch the "soaps."
3. Add stock and bring to boil, lower the heat, and simmer until vegetables are a bit softer but not mushy and have absorbed flavor from the stock. Turn off the heat.
4. Puree. If using a stand blender, remove soup from the pot, let cool, and puree it in the blender. Do this in batches if necessary.
5. Add liquid if the soup is too thick (slowly, so you don't get it too thin). Now is the time to use your culinary imagination by adding fresh herbs and spices to suit your taste buds (see spice chart on page 166). Simmer slowly another five to ten minutes to blend flavors.
6. Ladle into bowls, garnish, serve, and enjoy!

Once you have mastered this basic procedure, the only limit is your imagination. If your imagination is lacking, there are endless Web sites with delicious recipes. Those calling for a dollop of cream can be made just as tasty by substituting a dollop of nonfat yogurt. Greek yogurt is a great substitute for sour cream, as it is creamier and thicker than plain yogurt.

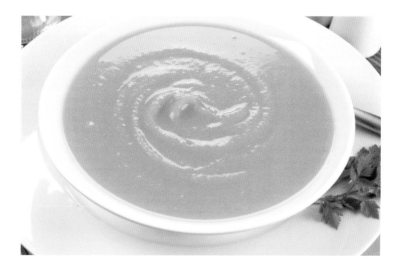

Here are some simple techniques for preparing and cooking a variety of vegetables. After the general prep, proceed to step two or three (page 162) as desired. You can also prepare more vegetables than you will need for your soup and freeze them for future use. In that case, you would just puree the excess amount separately. If you're making extra puree to use at a later time, blend for about two minutes. With some vegetables you will need to add a few teaspoons of water to get a smoother, creamier texture.

BEETS

PREP
Leave them whole and unpeeled. Trim any stems to 1 inch. Wrap in aluminum foil.

COOK
Roast at 400° F for about 1 hour. If beets can be pierced with a fork, they are ready. Remove from oven, cool to touch, then peel, chop, and add to stock. Another way to prepare beets is to cook them in a double boiler or pressure cooker until tender.

You can also peel them raw (be sure to wear gloves and peel them on plastic wrap, since they will stain your hands and other surfaces). Add them to the stock to simmer with everything else so that you don't have to dirty more dishes. Remember, the intense reddishness in beets will color your soup.

BUTTERNUT SQUASH, ACORN SQUASH, PUMPKIN

PREP
Cut off the stem, cut squash in half lengthwise, and scrape out seeds.

COOK
Place halves flesh-side down on a cookie sheet. Cover with foil and roast at 400° F for 45 to 50 minutes. Scoop out the flesh and add to stock. You can also peel the squash, add it to the stock, and let it simmer along with the other ingredients until tender.

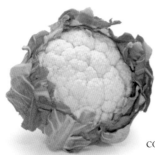

CAULIFLOWER

PREP
Cut off florets and discard core.

COOK
Steam for 8 to 10 minutes then add to stock, or add directly to the stock and cook 10 to 15 minutes.

BROCCOLI

PREP
Cut off florets and peel the stems with a vegetable peeler. Cut the stems into manageable pieces and add to your mix. You will get more for your money and the stems will add texture.

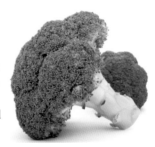

COOK
Steam for 6 to 7 minutes. The florets should be tender and bright green. Watch them closely so you don't overcook them to an olive color. Add the broccoli florets to the stock just before blending to be sure they don't overcook. You can also add the broccoli to the stock and cook.

CARROTS

PREP
Peel, trim the ends, and cut into 3-inch chunks.

COOK
Steam separately for 10 to 12 minutes or add directly to the stock.

MUSHROOMS

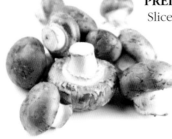

PREP
Slice mushrooms (or purchase presliced).

COOK
Put a little oil in saucepan and sauté the mushrooms until soft, or you can add them toward the end of the cooking process.

SPINACH

PREP
Baby spinach will need no prep. For mature spinach, fold leaves in half lengthwise with the stem outside, and strip the stem off the leaf.

COOK
Steam or boil for 10 to 15 seconds or add at the end of the cooking process.

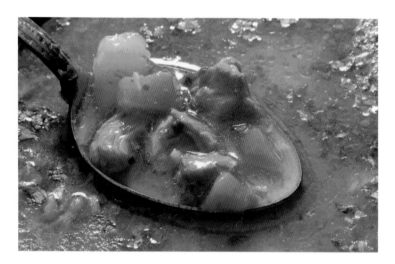

Soups with Stock

A stock soup is one of my favorites because of the mix-and-match ingredients you can use; my soups turn out different every time. All you need is a good stock, vegetables, spices, herbs, and some lean meat, if desired.

Start with the stock, add the vegetables with the longest cook times first, and then add those with shorter cook times. Meat may be precooked or cooked in the stock with the vegetables. Add the spices and herbs last. If you are not sure which ones to add, consult the chart on page 166. Try various combinations in little bowls of soup until you find the perfect blend.

Homemade soup stocks are well worth the effort. They add another dimension to soups that just plain water cannot achieve. Bouillon and boxed stocks are usually very high in sodium and can be expensive.

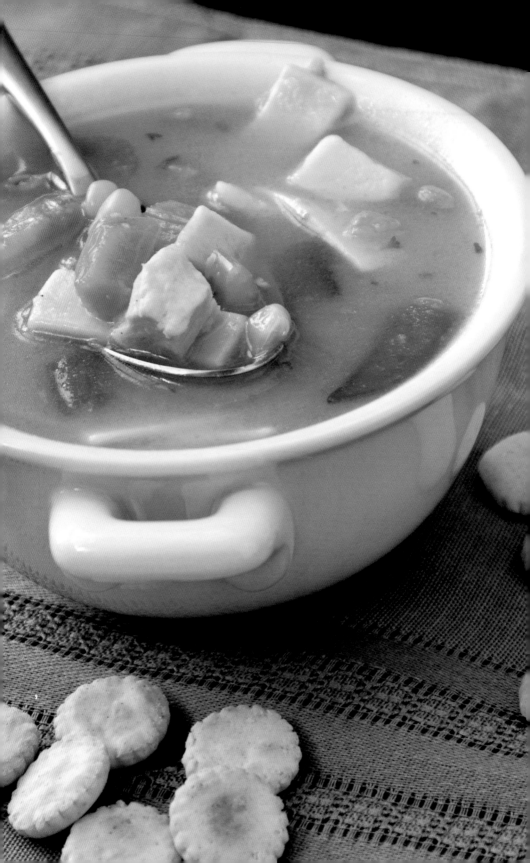

Making your own stock is not difficult and is definitely cheaper because you can make it from leftovers. Not only does it cost less, but it is tastier and more nutritious because of its fresh, natural ingredients.

Soup stock can be frozen in freezer bags of various sizes or in ice cube trays so the beginnings of a soup are always at your fingertips. This is another reason to invest in a large soup kettle if you don't already have one.

Roasted Chicken Stock

When making chicken stock, I use roasted rotisserie chicken. First, I strip the meat from the bones and freeze it in 3-ounce portions for later use. The bones also go into freezer bags. When I've accumulated bones from two to three chickens, I thaw them, oven roast for additional flavor, and make up a large batch of stock.

To make the stock, place the bones in a large pot and cover with water. Prepare the vegetables by washing them thoroughly. Don't peel the carrots, just scrub, slice in 1-inch rounds, and toss in the pot. Remove the outer layer of an onion and quarter it, leaving the root on for its nutrients and added flavor. Roughly chop celery, leaves and all. Add 2 cloves of mashed garlic and one medium bay leaf.

Let the pot simmer for 2 to 3 hours and then strain out the solids, leaving a delicious sodium-free broth. Refrigerate overnight and skim off any hardened fat. This broth, along with a few fresh vegetables, meat, and whole-wheat noodles, makes a soup that can't be beat.

Standard Chicken Stock

If you don't mind spending the extra time, your stock will have a deeper, fresher flavor if cooked using raw chicken. You can also use a combination of roasted chicken bones and fresh chicken backs and necks (prepackaged or requested from your butcher).

The process is the same as for Roasted Chicken Stock, except that a foam may rise to the top. Keep the heat low and skim off the foam.

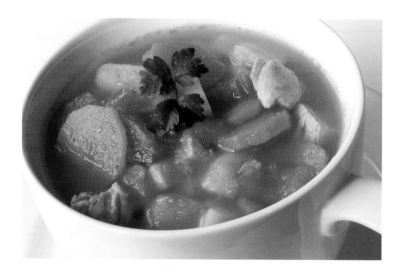

Turkey Stock

Follow the same directions as for Roasted Chicken Stock, except one turkey carcass will make a sizable batch of stock. After deboning and portioning the meat, you can freeze the carcass until ready to make your stock.

Brown Beef Broth

Start with 3 to 4 pounds of raw beef bones. The shank, neck, knuckle, leg bones, and oxtail work best. You can ask your butcher to cut them into smaller pieces.

Most vegetables or dry herbs will add flavor to a stock, but base flavors are carrots, celery, and onions. Avoid strongly flavored vegetables such as cabbage and broccoli.

The combinations I prefer to use in my beef broth: 2 onions, un-peeled and quartered; 2 to 3 large carrots, roughly chopped; 2 to 3 celery ribs, roughly chopped (include leaves); a few sprigs of fresh thyme (1 teaspoon dried); 2 bay leaves; and 10 peppercorns, lightly crushed (4 allspice berries can be substituted, if desired).

(1) Place the bones in a roasting pan in a 450° F oven for 20 to 30 minutes, turning occasionally until bones are slightly browned. (2) Add onions, carrots, and celery. Roast for 30 minutes more;

baste bones and vegetables 2 or 3 times with juice which accumulates during roasting. (3) Transfer bones and vegetables to your stockpot. Pour off the fat from the roasting pan and discard. Add ½ to 1 cup water to the pan and bring to a boil. Stir, scrape browned bits from the roasting pan, and add the mixture to the stockpot. (4) Add about 18 to 20 cups of water, bring to a simmer, and skim frequently until all surface foam has been removed. (5) Add the rest of the ingredients; partially cover the stockpot and simmer 4 to 6 hours. (6) Strain stock through a colander, then refrigerate overnight to let fat rise to the surface. (7) Skim off all the fat, and the stock is ready to use.

Vegetable Stock

This stock can be used for all vegetarian soups, as well as meat, poultry, and fish soups.

1) Roughly chop and add to a large stockpot 3 to 4 large celery ribs, 1 large quartered onion, 2 slices ginger root, 1 large yellow bell pepper, 1 parsnip, mushroom stems, and tomato peelings, followed by 2 tablespoons light soy sauce, 3 bay leaves, a handful of parsley sprigs, 3 sprigs fresh thyme, 1 sprig fresh rosemary, and 8 to 10 ground black peppercorns. (2) Cover with 15 to 16 cups of cold water. Bring slowly to a boil, lower heat, and simmer for 30 to 40 minutes, stirring occasionally. (3) Allow to cool. Strain, and then discard vegetables. This stock is ready for immediate use.

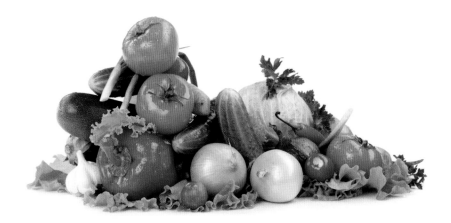

The following charts give suggestions for vegetables, lean meats, herbs, and spices that work well for stock soups:

Vegetables for Soups

Artichokes	Buy canned artichoke hearts packed in water and cut to the size that you desire.
Asparagus	Cut off the base of the stems, to about halfway up, and cut into bite-size pieces.
Bean sprouts	Add at the end of cooking process; stir in and serve immediately.
Beans, green	Cut into bite-size pieces and place in double boiler to steam until tender, then run under cold water to stop cooking process. Store on the countertop or in the refrigerator until ready. Add at the end of the cooking process.
Beets	Peel, chop roughly, julienne, or coarsely grate. There are not many soup recipes that call for beets, and how they are prepared and added differ, but they do take longer to cook, depending on size.
Broccoli	Cut off florets and slice stems into thin pieces. Add to the soup the last 3 minutes of cook time to prevent overcooking.
Brussels sprouts	Halve or quarter and steam until tender. Add at the end of cook time.
Cabbage	Remove core and slice thinly. Add near end of cook time. I do not use red cabbage, as its color will bleed into the stock.
Carrots	Peel, cut into bite-size pieces, or dice. Add early in the cooking process, as they take more time to cook.
Cauliflower	Cut into bite-size pieces and add when you have 3 minutes' cooking time remaining.
Celery	Remove base, leaves, and yellow stalk. Cut into bite-size pieces or dice. Best when not overcooked.
Chard	Cut/shred into bite-size pieces and add near end of cook time.

Cilantro	Remove leaves from stem and mince finely. Add at the end of cook time.
Corn	Cut from the cob or buy frozen.
Cucumbers	Buy English cucumbers and dice or slice. Peel regular cucumbers, remove seeds, and then dice or slice.
Eggplant	Remove outside skin and dice into bite-size pieces. Add near the end of cook time.
Garlic	Remove outside paper skin. Mince and sweat in covered saucepan for fuller flavor, or add directly to soup, or slice off top section and place on saucepan, cut-side down, and roast in the oven for 20 minutes at 350° F. Remove from the oven and allow it to rest for 5 minutes or until cool enough to touch. Squeeze out the meat and add to the soup.
Ginger	Peel with a spoon and use a cheese grater to shred.
Greens	Cut into bite-size pieces.
Kale	Blanch (place in boiling water for 1 minute and remove to cold water). Slice into bite-size pieces.
Kohlrabi	Peel outside layer and add early to the soup, as it requires more cook time.
Onions, green	Slice into bite-size pieces. Add white section at the beginning and green at the end of cook time.
Onions: red, yellow, white	Remove outer skin and slice or dice into bite-size pieces. Brown in a pan after meats.
Peas, sugar	Cut into bite-size pieces and add at the end of cook time.
Peppers: green, red, yellow, and orange	Remove core and seeds. Dice or slice into bite-size pieces. Roast, slice, and add to the soup at the end. Adds a piquant flavor.

Potatoes	Option 1: Peel and cut into bite-size pieces. Option 2: Scrub well, don't peel, and cut into bite-size pieces.

Add half-way through cook time since they take longer but will become mushy if overcooked. |
Rutabagas	Discard outside layer, cut into bite-size pieces, and add to stock early, as they will take more time to cook.
Spinach	Add at the end of cook time.
Squash, acorn	Quarter and bake or steam until soft; remove from the shell. Adding this to soups makes them creamier.
Squash, butternut and spaghetti	Peel and cut into bite-size pieces. Add early to the stock.
Squash, summer and zucchini	Slice and grill, or dice into bite-size pieces. Cooks in a short amount of time.
Sweet potatoes and yams	Peel and cut into bite-size pieces. Add early to stock.
Tomatoes	Dice and add at the end of cook time.
Turnips	Peel and cut into bite-size pieces. Add half-way through cook time.
Water chestnuts	Buy sliced canned and add. Do not need a lot of time to cook but will add a surprisingly nice texture to the soup.

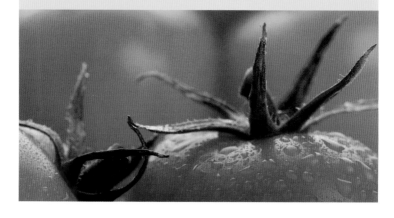

Types of Meats	Preparing Meats for Soups
Leftover lean meats	Note: Leftover meats from previous meals make excellent additions to soups.
Chicken	
White meat	The easiest way is to buy a roasted chicken, debone, and freeze meat or use immediately. Chicken breasts can be grilled, pan-fried, or baked. There are numerous recipes calling for cooked chicken. You can also roast a whole chicken in the oven or braise it in your slow cooker.
Beef	
Extra-lean beef	Brown in skillet then package in desired quantities. I usually add onions, garlic, and spices. When I want taco soup, I just pull out a bag and add the meat to the rest of the ingredients.
Eye of round	Roast in oven. After it cools, cut into desired portions and package for freezing. I use a smaller bag for myself, but if I'm preparing for a group, I take out an extra bag or two.
Flank	Grill and use leftovers for soup. Most soups, such as vegetable beef soup, call for small meat chunks.
Rump roast	Roast in oven or braise in slow cooker.
Pork	
Pork sirloin	Roast bite-size pieces in oven or braise in slow cooker. Cool and cut up for soups such as Miso or Sweet and Sour Pork Soup. I add this to pork noodles (whole-wheat, of course).

Fish	Fish is fairly expensive, so I buy mostly fillets. Watch for sales, especially on shrimp, which can be used in several delicious soups (gumbos) in smaller amounts than required for an entree. Cod and haddock are cheaper and can be broiled or baked then cut into chunks for chowders. Buy big and freeze the extra for later use. Fish cooks quickly and can be added raw toward the end of the cook time.
Lamb	Lamb is also an expensive option, but if you love chops and shanks, you can usually find them in your meat department. They can be fried (chops) or roasted (shanks) then deboned. Ground lamb can also be used for Lamb Kubbeh (dumpling) that is dropped into a tasty vegetable soup.

Spice Chart

Types of Flavors	Spice	Spice Blend from NutriFit
Latin/ Mexican	Cumin, cilantro, onion, lime	Calypso blend
Asian	Ginger, garlic, sesame oil, soy sauce (reduced salt), anise	
Thai	Cilantro, basil, lemon, peanut butter (reduced calorie, used sparingly)	
Barbecue	Chili powder, garlic, onion, liquid smoke	
Southwest	Cilantro, onion, jalapeño, tomato, lime	Calypso blend
Seafood	Lemon, pepper	Lemon Garden blend
Holidays	Orange, cinnamon, nutmeg	Certainly Cinnamon blend
Indian	Curry	Rockin' Moroccan blend
Italian	Basil, oregano, thyme	Mediterranean blend
Spanish	Tomatoes, olive oil, olives	French Riviera blend

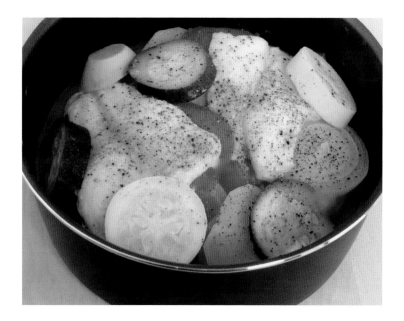

Recipes for Soups

Layered Fish Stew

1 tablespoon canola oil
1 medium onion, thinly sliced
2 cloves garlic, minced
3 fresh tomatoes, sliced
1 potato, peeled and thinly sliced
1 to 1½ pounds of any firm white fish fillets (such as cod)
2 zucchini or yellow squash, sliced
½ teaspoon salt
¼ teaspoon pepper
½ cup water

Oil bottom of a lidded pot. Layer one-half of each of the ingredients: onion, garlic, tomatoes, potato, fish, zucchini or yellow squash, salt, pepper, and water. Repeat in the same order with remaining ingredients. Simmer, covered, for 45 minutes. Serves 4.

Guida Ponte

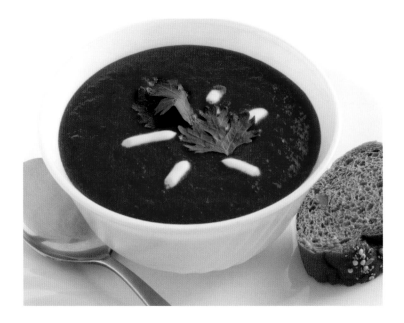

Beet Soup

1 tablespoon olive oil
1 small onion, chopped
2 cloves garlic, whole
4 medium to large beets, cut in large chunks
1 teaspoon brown sugar
2 teaspoons red wine vinegar
4 cups chicken broth
Salt and pepper to taste
2 tablespoons nonfat or Greek yogurt
Cilantro (optional)

Heat oil in heavy stockpot over medium heat; add onion, garlic, and beets. Stir in brown sugar and red wine vinegar. Add chicken broth and bring to a boil. Let simmer over medium heat until beets are soft. Remove from heat, cool, and spoon into blender; blend until smooth. Add salt and pepper to taste. When ready to serve, top with a dollop of yogurt. Serve hot or chilled. Serves 4.

Guida Ponte

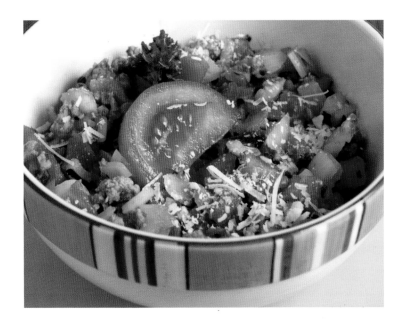

Mexican Soup

1 teaspoon olive oil
1 small onion, diced
4 ounces lean beef or turkey, ground
½ cup celery, diced
½ cup hominy
½ cup medium–hot picante sauce or spiced salsa
2 tablespoons cilantro, chopped
2 tablespoons hard cheese, grated, such as Parmesan (Cotija)
1 tomato wedge (optional)

Heat oil in saucepan. Add onion and brown, then add meat and brown. Add celery, hominy, and picante sauce and simmer 5 to 10 minutes. Top with cilantro and cheese to serve. Serves 1.

Note: Hard cheese, such as Parmesan or Cotija, is more flavorful than soft, thus you do not need to use as much.

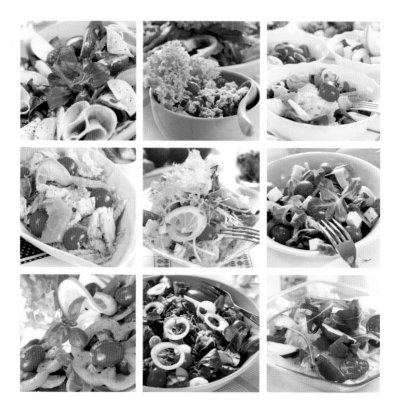

Salads

Salads can be your best friend when you're trying to lose weight. Cool and crunchy and packed with lots of nutrients, they can be a great accompaniment to an entree or a satisfying meal by themselves.

Too often our limited concept of salads begins and ends with lettuce. There are so many different combinations of vegetables, fruits, beans, and grains that can give your salad a special twist.

Dressings can be the downfall of many a healthy salad. For instance, a 2-tablespoon serving of many dressings may have as many as 150 calories, with a high percent coming from fat. Look for flavorful low-fat dressings such as Newman's Own Lighten Up Low Fat Sesame Ginger. It adds a lot of flavor for 35 calories per 2 tablespoons but is a little high in sodium. Omit soft cheeses, bacon bits, and nuts, as these tend to be high in calories.

Guidelines for Salads
Salad Bar

Salads are easier to make than ever because greens are available from the grocery store already cleaned and snipped into bite-size pieces. (The USDA still recommends rinsing bagged salad greens as a precaution.)

Packaged salads include:

1. Baby spinach
2. Cole slaw mix
3. Caesar salad mix
4. European mix
5. Iceberg mix
6. Romaine mix
7. Spring greens (my favorite)

Suggested salad mix-ins:

1. Artichoke hearts (without oil)
2. Green olives (sparingly, 4 olives per serving)
3. Black olives (sparingly, 4 olives per serving)
4. Hard-cooked eggs (1 per serving)
5. Grated hard cheese (sparingly, 1 to 2 tablespoons)
6. Chicken breast (3 ounces per serving)
7. Radishes
8. Asparagus
9. Jicama
10. Bell peppers
11. Celery
12. Mushrooms
13. Sprouts
14. Snap peas
15. Three-bean salad
16. Berries
17. Apples
18. Tuna
19. Oranges or Clementines
20. Avocado (¼ per serving)

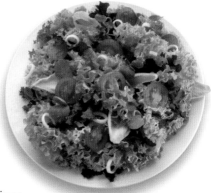

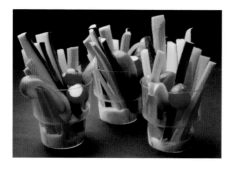

Stand-Up Salad

1 small paper or plastic
    cup
2 tablespoons of your
    favorite lite dressing
Vegetable strips (celery,
    carrots, jicama, snap
    peas, bell peppers,
    etc.)

Place your favorite low-fat dressing in the bottom of a cup, and
then stand the vegetables in the dip. When you're ready to eat
them, the vegetables are already dipped.

Walking Salad

1 apple
1 tablespoon pineapple or lemon juice
1 tablespoon reduced calorie peanut butter
    combined with 1 tablespoon raisins

Slice off top of the apple. Hollow out the core, leaving the bottom
of the apple intact. Brush hollow with pineapple or lemon juice.
Fill with peanut butter and raisin mixture. Replace top of apple and
place in sandwich bag until ready to eat.

This is excellent for hikes or walks. It gives you that extra energy
to keep you going.

Garbanzo Salad

1 (15-ounce) can garbanzo beans, drained and rinsed
1 small sweet onion, diced
¼ cup fresh parsley or cilantro, minced
3 tablespoons lite vinaigrette dressing

In a salad bowl, combine garbanzo beans, onion, and parsley or
cilantro. Add dressing. Serving size is ½ cup. Serves 4.

Fresh Garden Salad

1 bunch asparagus, steamed
¼ cup onion, minced
1 cup zucchini, cut into thin matchstick strips
1 cup carrots, cut into thin matchstick strips
3 tablespoons lite vinaigrette dressing

In a salad bowl, combine asparagus, onion, zucchini, and carrots. Add dressing, as desired. Serves 4 to 6.

Sliced Beet Salad

1 head Romaine lettuce, chopped, or bag of spinach
2 (15-ounce) cans sliced pickled beets, drained
4 green onions, sliced
2 hard-cooked eggs, sliced
¼ cup lite vinaigrette dressing

On a large platter, arrange lettuce or spinach and add beets. Decorate with green onions and egg slices and drizzle with vinaigrette. Serves 6 to 8.

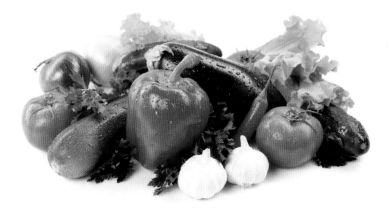

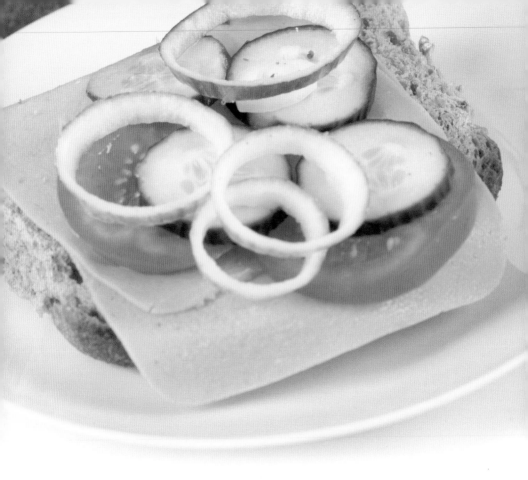

Sandwiches and Wraps

Sandwiches are fast, simple, and portable. I always use whole-grain breads, flatbreads, and wraps for my sandwiches. To cut costs, I buy day-old whole-wheat bread then divide the loaf into 2-slice portions and freeze in Ziploc bags. When I'm ready to eat, I brush off any ice crystals and toast the bread before making a sandwich.

I occasionally use Flat Out Healthy Grain Low-Fat Wraps and whole-wheat Bagel Thins. I also buy Oroweat rounds and 6-inch corn tortillas, which are 40 to 60 calories each.

These quick-to-fix, fun-to-eat sandwiches, wraps, and pocket sandwiches are perfect for lunches whether you're on the go or at home.

Vegetables for Sandwiches, Wraps, and Pocket Sandwiches

Artichokes	Buy canned artichoke hearts packed in water and cut into slices to use on sandwich, wrap, or pocket sandwich.
Asparagus	Cut off the base of the stems. Either grill or steam and then place on sandwich, wrap, or pocket sandwich.
Bean sprouts	Place on sandwich, wrap, or pocket sandwich.
Cabbage	Shred and place on sandwich, wrap, or pocket sandwich.
Carrots	Grate and place on sandwich, wrap, or pocket sandwich, or serve as a side.
Celery	Chop and add to a sandwich filling or serve as a side.
Chard	Remove hard part of stem and place on sandwich, wrap, or pocket sandwich.
Cilantro	Remove leaves from stem and mince or place whole leaves on sandwich, wrap, or pocket sandwich for a flavor boost.
Cucumbers	Slice and use on sandwich, wrap, or pocket sandwich.
Garlic	Slice the top off a head of garlic and brush with olive oil. Wrap in foil and place on a baking sheet and bake for 20 minutes at 350° F. Squeeze out the meat and add as a spread on sandwich, wrap, or pocket sandwich.
Ginger	Finely grate and add a little to a sandwich filling.
Greens	Add leaves to add texture to a sandwich, wrap, or pocket sandwich.
Onions, green	Cut in half and place on top of sandwich, wrap, or pocket sandwich.
Onions, sweet or red	Thinly slice sweet or red onions and place on sandwich, wrap, or pocket sandwich.

Peas, sugar	Enjoy the crunch this adds to a sandwich, wrap, or pocket sandwich.
Peppers: green, red, yellow and orange	Slice thinly and place on sandwich, wrap, or pocket sandwich.
Potatoes	Thinly slice leftover potatoes, sprinkle with a little seasoning, and enjoy in a sandwich.
Spinach	Place leaves on sandwich, wrap, or pocket sandwich.
Squash, summer and zucchini	Slice, brush with olive oil, and season with salt, pepper, and herbs as desired. Place on a sandwich, or slice, dice, and place on a wrap or pocket sandwich.
Tomatoes	Slice and place on sandwich or dice for a wrap or pocket sandwich.
Water chestnuts	Buy canned sliced water chestnuts and place on sandwich, wrap, or pocket sandwich to add flavor and crunch.

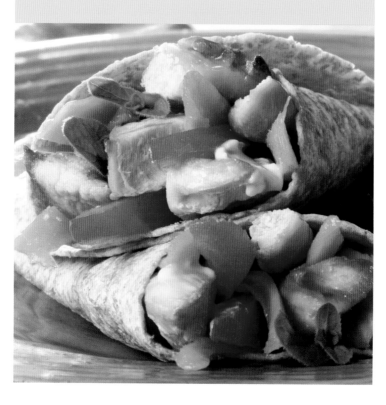

Sandwich Meats

Type of Meat	Preparation Methods
Leftover lean meats	Leftover meats are ideal for sandwiches.
Chicken	
White meat	It's easiest to buy a roasted chicken, debone it, and use it for sandwiches, wraps, or pocket sandwiches. What you don't use can be sliced and frozen. You can also grill chicken breasts and slice for sandwiches, wraps, or pocket sandwiches.
Beef	
Eye of round	Roast in oven or braise in slow cooker. Slice for sandwiches, wraps, or pocket sandwiches. Freeze remaining meat for future use.
Flank	Grill and use leftovers for sandwiches, wraps, or pocket sandwiches.
Rump roast	Roast in oven or braise in slow cooker. Slice and place on sandwiches, wraps, or pocket sandwiches. Freeze remaining meat for future use.
Pork	
Pork sirloin	Roast in oven or cook in slow cooker. Slice or shred and place on sandwiches, wraps, or pocket sandwiches. Freeze remaining meat for future use.
Fish	Grill or broil for sandwiches, or tear into smaller pieces for wraps or pocket sandwiches.

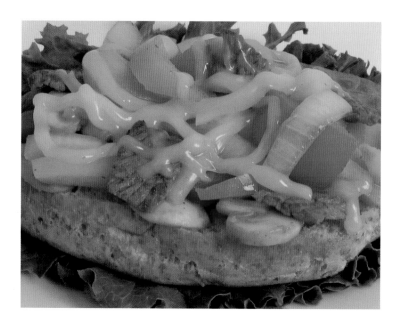

Steak Sandwich

½ tablespoon olive oil
1 small onion, diced
4 ounces lean steak, thinly sliced
5 small sweet bell peppers or ½ large bell pepper
½ cup mushrooms, sliced
½ large whole-wheat roll
2 tablespoons hard cheese, grated

In a skillet heat oil. Add onions and cook until tender. Add steak and cook until browned. Add peppers and sauté, then add mushrooms and cook until done. Place on roll and top with grated cheese. Serves 1.

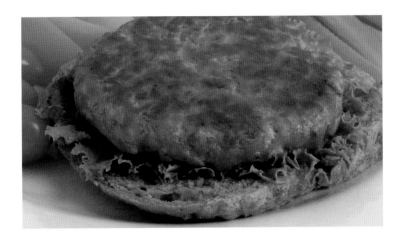

Turkey Burgers

One pound of ground turkey provides 4 servings. Check the fat content, as ground turkey sold in tubes usually has a higher fat content.

1 pound lean ground turkey
1 egg
½ medium onion, chopped
Seasoning of your choice
½ large whole-wheat roll per serving

In a bowl mix ground turkey, egg, and onion. Add seasoning. Shape into 4 patties. Grill or cook in a frying pan until browned on bottom; flip over. Cover the pan with a lid and turn off the heat to allow turkey to continue to cook. Serves 4.

Note: I usually prepare ground turkey by dividing a pound into 4 equal portions, forming them into patties, placing them in Ziploc bags, and freezing. Remove patties from the freezer and place in the refrigerator a day or two before you plan to use them.

Toppings might include:
    Roasted peppers
    Grilled or chopped onions
    Raw spinach leaves
    Lettuce
    Tomatoes
    Chopped red or green bell peppers

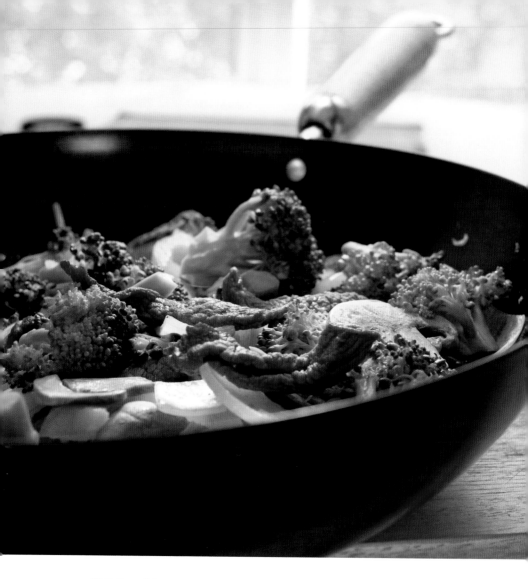

Stir-Fry

Stir-fry is easy to prepare, and the combinations are endless. You can vary the flavor with spices, or you can change the meats and vegetables you use. You can make a specific stir-fry recipe or look in your refrigerator and assess what will go together for your dish. It's the next best thing to soup in the number of varieties and ways it can be made. There is really no wrong way to combine stir-fry ingredients.

1. Clean and prepare the vegetables. If they take a long time to cook, you may choose to precook. I prepare my vegetables in small bowls and then line them up in the order that I will put them into the stir-fry. Add the vegetables that will cook longest first.

2. If you want marinated meats: Place prepared meat in a Ziploc bag. Add half the marinade (reserve the other half for later), seal the bag, and refrigerate 20 to 30 minutes (place it in a bowl, just in case the bag leaks).

3. Drain the meat, discard the marinade, and fry the meat in a little heated canola oil. Remove from pan and set aside. If you are using precooked, skip this step and add the meat at the end of the cooking process. When meat is ready, remove from pan and cook the vegetables.

4. Add prepared vegetables to the hot pan (may need a little oil) in the order of their required cooking time. Stir constantly until the vegetables are just barely tender (there is a reason it's called stir-fry). Now add the meat to the vegetables.

5. Add sauce to the pan and stir. If you need a thicker sauce, make it with 2 tablespoons cornstarch and 2 tablespoons cold water, stirring out all lumps. Add to reserved marinade or marinade that you want to thicken. Pour over meat and vegetables and stir just until bubbling hot and thickened. Serve.

Stir-Fry Vegetables

Artichokes	Buy canned artichoke hearts packed in water. Drain and pat dry so they don't splatter, and add at the end of cook time to heat through.
Asparagus	Cut off the base of the stems, and cut into bite-size pieces.
Bean sprouts	Add at the end of cook time, stir in, and serve immediately.

Beans, green	Cut into 2- to 3-inch lengths and add to the stir-fry first, as they take longer to cook. Cook till crisp and a little tender and still bright green.
Broccoli	Cut off florets and slice stems into thin pieces. Add to the stir-fry near the end so it doesn't overcook. In China I have seen them steam the broccoli and add it to stir-fry at the very end. Don't overcook to an olive color!
Brussels sprouts	Cut into halves or quarters and steam until tender. Add at the end of cook time. If you choose not to precook, add first, as they take longer to cook.
Cabbage	Remove core and slice thinly. Add near end of cook time.
Carrots	Peel and cut into thick julienne-style slices or cut crosswise at an angle. Add early in the cooking process, as they take more time. If you prefer carrots on the tender side, steam them and add them to the stir-fry just before serving.
Cauliflower	Cut into bite-size pieces and add midway or near the end of cook time.
Celery	Remove base, leaves, and yellow stalk. Cut into bite-size pieces or 2-inch strips.
Chard	Cut into bite-size pieces and add near the end of cook time.
Cilantro	Remove leaves from stem and mince finely. Add at the end of cook time.
Corn	Fresh corn should be blanched and cut from the cob, but frozen corn works just as well. Toss in near the end of cook time.
Eggplant	Peel outside skin with a knife. Cut into thick julienne slices and add near the end of cook time.

Garlic	Remove papery outside skin. Mince and sauté in a little peanut or canola oil at the beginning of the stir-fry. Make sure the oil is not too hot or the garlic will burn.
Ginger	Peel with a spoon and use a cheese grater to shred. I often prepare ginger ahead of time then freeze in very small portions.
Greens	Cut into bite-size pieces and cook for a short time. In China they have so many greens that they will often combine them into a stir-fry all by themselves.
Onions, green	Remove outer peel and remove ends. Cut into 2- to 3-inch slices.
Onions: red, yellow, white	Remove outer peel and slice or dice into bite-size pieces (I prefer slices). Add with other vegetables.
Peas, sugar	Cut into bite-size pieces and add near the end of cook time.
Peppers: green, red, yellow, and orange	Cut in half, remove core and seeds, and slice lengthwise. Add with onions and garlic.
Spinach	Coarsely chop and add at the end of cook time.
Squash, summer and zucchini	Wash and cut into halves or thirds, and slice into thin wedges or rounds.
Tomatoes	Dice or cut in wedges and add at the end of cook time.
Water chestnuts	Buy canned sliced and add near the end of cook time to provide a nice crunchy texture.

Types of Meats	Preparing Meats for Stir-Fry
Leftover lean meats	Stir-fry is a great way to use leftover meat.
Chicken	
White meat	Boneless skinless chicken breast is the easiest to prepare. Cut the breast into strips and place in marinade for 20 to 30 minutes (if one is being used). If not using marinade, fry strips in hot oil for 3 to 5 minutes, remove from heat, and add to cooked vegetables.
Beef	
Eye of round roast	Roast in oven or braise in slow cooker. If using fresh meat, cut across the grain into thin strips, marinate, and stir-fry for 6 to 8 minutes. Follow stir-fry instructions on page 181.
Flank	Grill and then use same procedure as above. If using fresh meat, cut across the grain into thin strips, marinate, and stir-fry for 6 to 8 minutes. Follow stir-fry instructions on page 181.
Rump roast	Roast in oven or braise in slow cooker. Use the same procedure as for eye of round roast. If fresh, follow stir-fry instructions on page 181.
Pork	
Pork tenderloin	Roast in the oven or braise in slow cooker. Cool and cut in strips, put in freezer bags, and label, date, and freeze. If using fresh meat, cut across the grain into thin strips, marinate, and stir-fry for 6 to 8 minutes. Follow stir-fry instructions on page 181.
Fish	Fish is not a popular stir-fry ingredient, but if you're a big fish lover, precook fillets of your choice (shrimp is a tasty option). Cut fillets in strips then add last as fish tends to fall apart. Don't overcook shrimp. As soon as they turn pink, they are ready.
Lamb	Lamb can be very expensive. Use boneless lamb from the leg or loin. Cut into long 2-inch-wide strips along the grain of the meat, and then cut crosswise (across the grain) into thin slices. This better ensures tenderness. Follow stir-fry instructions on page 181.

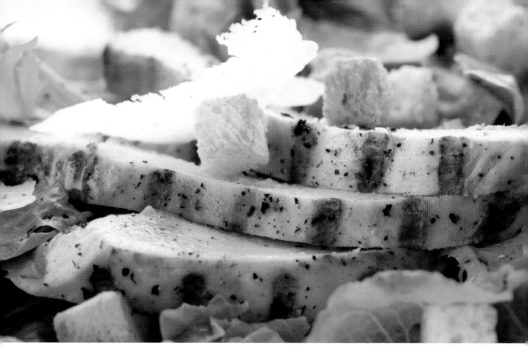

Main Dishes and One-Dish Meals

Main dishes are the foundation of your meal. It's especially handy when you can turn them into one-dish meals, since cooking everything in a single pot makes the prep work and clean-up that much easier.

So many of yesteryear's casseroles were heavy with cream-of-something soup and loads of starchy pasta or rice. For better health, incorporate more vegetables instead of starch and stay away from heavy sauces. You'll find your dishes are actually more full-flavored.

Red Cabbage, Onions, and Pork

½ tablespoon canola oil
1 small onion, diced
4 ounces lean pork loin or ground turkey
3 cups red cabbage, shredded
1 to 2 tablespoons mustard

Place oil in skillet and heat, then add onion and meat; brown. Add cabbage, and continue to cook. When ready to serve, top with mustard. Serves 1.

Mexican Ratatouille

1 tablespoon canola oil
1 onion, diced
1 pound lean ground beef or turkey
3 yellow squash, cut into bite-size pieces
2 to 3 medium tomatoes, diced
2 tablespoons cilantro, chopped
2 peppers (roasted peppers are suggested), any color
1 cup Pace Picante Sauce (medium spice if you want a little heat)
Add a little water if desired
1 tablespoon hard cheese per serving, grated

Place oil in a skillet and heat; add onions and meat and brown. Add squash and cook slightly. Add remaining ingredients except cheese and simmer until vegetables are tender. Place in a serving bowl and sprinkle with cheese. Serves 4.

Freeze-Ahead Meat Loaf

For extra vegetables in your diet
1 pound lean ground beef or turkey
1 carrot, grated
1 rib celery, diced
1 potato, grated
1 onion, diced
1 egg
2 tablespoons lite soy sauce
1 cup oatmeal (blend in blender until it becomes floury)
2 tablespoons mixed Italian seasoning or 1 teaspoon each of oregano, basil, and garlic powder plus dash of salt

Mix all ingredients well by hand. Place in bread pan that has been sprayed with cooking spray. Bake for 45 minutes at 350° F. Serves 5.

Portion leftovers into 4-ounce servings and place in Ziploc bags to freeze.

Bill Mansell

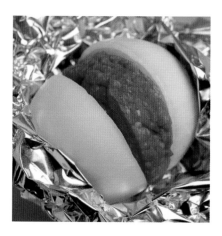

Meat Loaf in an Onion

4 large onions, peeled
  and halved
1 pound extra-lean
  ground beef or
  turkey
1 egg (optional)
¼ cup tomato sauce
  (optional)
½ teaspoon salt
⅛ teaspoon pepper

Remove the roots from the bottom ends of onions.

In a mixing bowl combine ground beef, egg, tomato sauce, salt, and pepper and mix by squeezing. Set aside.

Cut onions in half horizontally and remove center part of onion, leaving a ½ to ¾-inch-thick shell. (Save onion center for later use.) Divide meat mixture into 4 portions and roll into balls. Place meat mixture in the center of the 4 onion halves; put onions back together. Place onions in baking dish and bake in the oven at 350° F for 45 to 50 minutes. Serves 4.

Cooking on hot coals: I have demonstrated this favorite recipe outdoors for years. I like to have each person prepare their own and tend it on the charcoal or hot coals.

Prepare as directed above. Then place each onion in the center of a piece of 18-inch heavy-duty foil long enough to wrap around the onion, with 4 inches to spare on each side. Bring the foil ends together and roll down in small folds. Then flatten on both ends and roll in. Place on hot coals for 15 minutes on each side. Serves 4.

Frying Hamburgers, Steaks, or Fish

Try this method to cook meats such as hamburger or steak. Heat a skillet, add the meat, and turn it when browned. Sprinkle a little seasoning of your choice on top. Then turn the heat off, cover with a lid, and let the meat finish cooking.

With Fish: I follow the same steps as above but when the fish is turned, pour a little water in the pan, turn the heat off, and let the fish finish cooking with the steam heat.

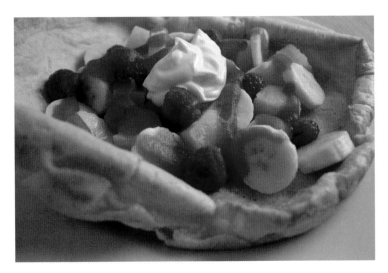

German Pancakes

Delicious for special occasions or for a holiday breakfast, this fluffy pancake should be eaten as soon as it comes out of the oven. You will need 4 pie tins for this recipe.

1 cup fat-free milk
1 cup all-purpose flour
6 large eggs
Dash salt
1 teaspoon vanilla
½ to 1 tablespoon butter (per pie tin)
Topping (see below)

Preheat oven to 400° F. Mix milk, flour, eggs, salt, and vanilla with an egg beater.

Put butter in the bottom of each pie and place in oven. Remove pans as soon as butter melts and tilt to grease entire pan.

Divide batter into each of the 4 pans. Bake 10 to 15 minutes, or until golden brown. The edges will puff up, and the pancake will form a well in the center. Spoon topping into the well, top with nonfat yogurt, and serve immediately. Serves 4.

Topping:
1 bag frozen raspberries, slightly thawed
1 can chunk pineapple, drained
2 bananas, sliced
½ cup nonfat or Greek yogurt

Spoon raspberries, pineapple, and bananas onto the pancakes and top with yogurt. (Total amount of fruit per serving should not exceed ¾ cup.)

Side Dishes

Side dishes can enhance a simple main course such as grilled chicken or fish. Give vegetables a starring role in your side dishes, because they add color to your plate. They're also a nutritional bargain because they cost you very little in calories. If your side dishes contain a starch, be sure to use whole-wheat pasta, brown rice, or another whole grain.

Vegetables

My main side dishes are usually vegetables. I eat them both raw and cooked. Cooked vegetables can be prepared in many different ways:

- Roasted in the oven. This is excellent for root vegetables and hard squashes.
- Grilled. Terrific for summer squashes, onions, and peppers.
- Steamed in double boiler. Excellent for all vegetables (90 percent of my vegetables are prepared this way).
- Frozen vegetables added to boiling water.

Pureed Squash

A favorite side or snack of mine is pureed squash. Quarter the squash and remove the seeds, place squash in the top of a double boiler, and steam until tender then scoop out of the shell. Place the squash into a food processor, or mash it with a potato masher. Add a little Smart Balance Light.

I place the pureed squash in 1-cup containers in the refrigerator to use throughout the week.

Pickled Beets

Pickled beets have a delicious tangy flavor and are a welcome addition to salads, side dishes, or snacks with ½ cup of nonfat cottage cheese.

6 beets
Flavored vinegar to cover beets

Clean and trim beets, leaving the roots intact. Place beets in top of a double boiler and steam cook (35 to 45 minutes); or cover with foil and roast in a 350° F degree oven 45 to 60 minutes or until fork tender. Cut the root and stem off, then peel and slice into quarter-inch slices. Place in a lidded container. Pour raspberry, pomegranate, or red wine vinegar over the beets until they are covered. Place the lid on the container and put it in the fridge for at least 3 days before eating. They will stay fresh in the fridge for up to 3 weeks. For a few calories, you'll enjoy a great taste.

Roasted Peppers

Roasted peppers add a unique flavor to such dishes as hamburgers, soups, and sides.

6 peppers, any color, large

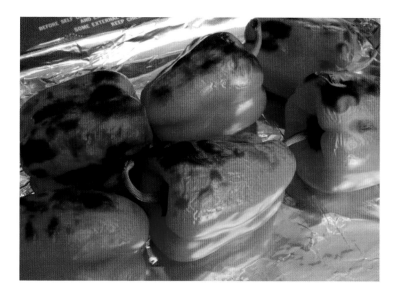

Place peppers on a foil-lined cookie sheet. Put them in the oven on the top rack, 3 inches from the broiler. Watch carefully as the peppers cook, turning them until all sides are roasted. Remove cookie sheet from the oven, and put the hot roasted peppers into a plastic bag to sweat. When cooled, take them out of the bag and remove the skins. Cut the peppers in half and remove the seeds. Place the halves in a plastic container and store covered in the fridge.

Desserts

In order to stay with a long-term program of healthy eating, you'll want a treat once in a while. I usually only have desserts on special occasions. But if your idea of dessert is a triple-size decadent concoction full of fudge, whipped cream, and so on, you will have to rethink the concept. Unfortunately, many desserts contain too much sugar, high-fructose corn syrup, white flour, hydrogenated oil, or saturated fat—and simply too many calories.

You don't have to swear completely off chocolate, though; studies have shown that having an occasional nibble of dark chocolate can be good for you. Dark chocolate contains antioxidants that fight high blood pressure and heart disease.

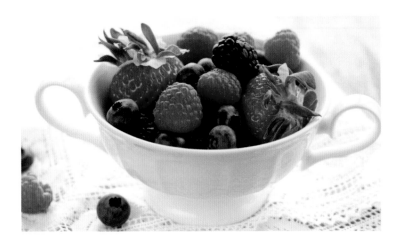

Fruit as Dessert

You may remember reading earlier in the book that a slice of watermelon or an orange is the only dessert I have seen served in China. When eating out with others who are having dessert, I always ask for a dish of fresh fruit.

Pineapple Dessert

1 tablespoon Smart Balance Light
1 slice pineapple packed in juice
1 teaspoon brown sugar

Melt Smart Balance Light in a small skillet. Top with pineapple slice and sprinkle with brown sugar. Cook until bottom of pineapple is golden brown and sugar is melted. Serves 1.

Jackie Keller

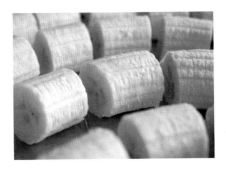

Banana Shake

When milk shakes and malts became no-nos in my food program, I began to look for replacements. Here is a delicious substitute for high-calorie milk shakes. Let a bunch of bananas ripen until there are a just few brown spots. Peel, cut them in 1-inch sections, and freeze in Ziploc bags until ready to make your shake (1 banana per bag).

1 frozen banana, prepared as described above
1½ cups 8th Continent Soy Milk or skimmed milk
½ teaspoon vanilla

Place all ingredients in a blender and blend until smooth and creamy. One serving is under 200 calories.

Fruit Shake: You can use other fruit to make similar shakes. If I don't eat soft fruit, such as peaches and nectarines, within a few days, I peel them and cut them into 1-inch pieces, place them on a piece of plastic wrap on a tray, and freeze them uncovered. When frozen, I divide the pieces into serving portions and package them into Ziploc sandwich bags. Remove as much air from the bag as possible before sealing it. When you're ready for a shake, use the above ingredients and directions, substituting other fruit for part or all of the banana.

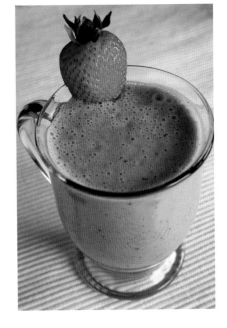

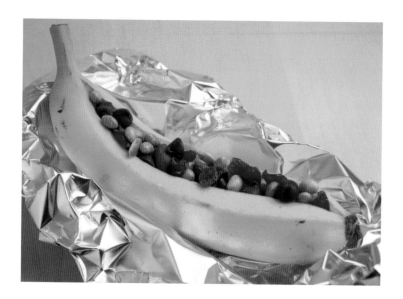

Banana Boat

While visiting China, I learned how to prepare some Chinese dishes at the home of our guide, and I was asked if I had an American dish I might want to show them. All I had with me was my snack pack of dark chocolate pieces, dried cranberries, and soy nuts. On the table I saw bananas, and the idea occurred to me to use what I'd brought to make a banana-boat dessert.

2 tablespoons dark chocolate pieces
2 tablespoons dried cranberries
2 tablespoons soy nuts
2 bananas

Mix together chocolate pieces, cranberries, and soy nuts. Cut a slit lengthwise about two-thirds of the way through each unpeeled banana from stem to base. Open the banana so that it looks like a canoe. Fill the slit with half of the snack mix. Repeat with second banana. Wrapped in foil in their skins, cook bananas over hot coals or in the oven at 350° F. If microwaving, cover them with plastic wrap and cook until the chocolate is melted. Serves 2.

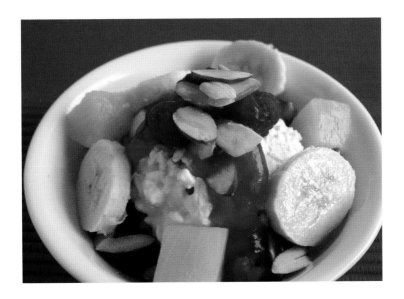

Cottage Cheese Sundae

When I get a hankering for an ice cream sundae treat, this is what I make! It's just a half cup of nonfat cottage cheese topped with ½ small banana, ⅓ cup of pineapple chunks, ½ cup of raspberries, and a tablespoon of slivered almonds.

Preserving Foods

A helpful book to buy or borrow if you are going to preserve foods is the *Ball Blue Book Guide to Preserving.*

From my kitchen window I can see squirrels running from one yard to another, gathering food. In the fall, small dried apples that have dropped from the tree seem to be the preference of the day.

During autumn, I begin to feel like the squirrels in the backyard. On Saturdays, I frequent the farmers' markets, bringing home boxes of produce to put away for winter. As a small child I would watch my mother bottle peaches, pears, and applesauce. My parents told me that when they were young, they would have gone hungry if they hadn't preserved their harvests in the fall.

I do likewise. I'll roast garden-fresh tomatoes, onions, and garlic in the oven to make a tomato-based sauce. After removing the roasted vegetables from the oven, I let them cool and then puree them in the blender. On the stove they cook down until a thick tomato sauce forms that I can freeze and use later for spaghetti, chili, or tomato soup. I'll add the spices later when I decide how I am going to use the sauce (see recipe on page 197).

Inside some metal cabinets in the garage, I squirrel away butternut squash, onions, apples, and potatoes in closed cardboard boxes. Stored in this way, the food doesn't freeze in the winter, and keeps for about two months. This works particularly well in cooler climates.

My dehydrator gets a workout when I make apple chips for my snacks. They also make welcome holiday gifts for friends and neighbors.

This winter preparation is part of my pioneer heritage and a way of life. As we gather around the dinner table, we give thanks for the food, the hardworking people who raised it, and the blessings of being able to store it. We benefit greatly from the health benefits that come from home-grown, home-stored, and home-prepared food.

Home Canning

Home canning and freezing are good ways to have nutritious food products on hand. Fresh, quality produce preserves well for later use. It's even better when you are able to grow your own.

Be sure to follow a reputable canning guide to avoid food safety issues. It's best to follow a tested recipe from a trusted source, such as the USDA's Extension Services or the *Ball Blue Book Guide to Preserving*.

Fruits that are high in acid such as peaches, pears, and other soft fruits are good candidates for water-bath canning, while low-acid vegetables, such as corn and green beans, must be canned using a pressure canner.

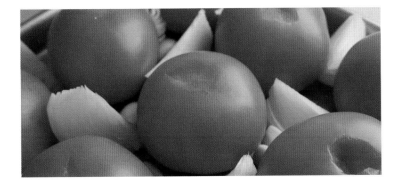

Light and Lean Tomato Sauce

One of my favorite times of the year is when the tomatoes begin to ripen. I love locally grown tomatoes, because they can be fixed in so many ways and are readily available.

Here's a recipe for a light, lean tomato sauce made from fresh tomatoes and frozen in canning jars.

The best part of cooking my own food is that I know the quality of the tomatoes, onions, and garlic that go into the sauce. There are no hidden fillers, fats, sugar, or corn syrup in my sauce.

15 tomatoes
2 large onions, peeled and quartered
5 cloves garlic

Cover a large rimmed baking sheet with heavy-duty foil. Cut the stems from 15 tomatoes (I use medium or large) and place them cut-side down on the tray, leaving about ½ inch between them to allow for hot air circulation.

Make a small cross on what is now the top of each tomato. Add two large peeled and quartered onions and five cloves of garlic to the baking sheet and place it in a 350° F oven. Let the vegetables roast until the tomatoes are softened and their skins slip off.

Remove the tray from the oven and let the vegetables cool for a few minutes, then skin the tomatoes with a pair of tongs, if desired.

Place all of the vegetables into a blender and process. Pour the mixture into a large, heavy saucepan and simmer at a low temperature, stirring occasionally, until the tomatoes have thickened to the consistency of a spaghetti sauce. This may take several hours.

You can add your favorite seasonings now, or wait until you determine the sauce's use. The intensity of some herbs change during storage, so go a little light with the seasonings until you are sure you will get just the intensity you want.

Remove the thickened sauce from the range and allow it to cool. Pour into pint or quart jars. Fill the jars to within ¾ of an inch of the top and freeze. Don't put the lids on yet or the jar might break when the sauce expands during freezing. Put the lids and rings on after the sauce is frozen. The sauce will last one year in the freezer.

Thaw in the refrigerator and use in your favorite tomato-based dish.

Guida Ponte

Dry It, You'll Like It

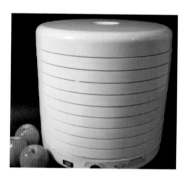

Drying is the oldest method of preserving food. Ancient peoples didn't have refrigerators, freezers, tin cans, or jars. They simply used the sun to dry berries and meat for jerky.

Today, drying still has advantages. If you come back from a farmer's market with a bushel of tomatoes or you have a tree in your backyard loaded with fruit, you can shrink down most of that inventory into a few containers. As the food dries, its natural sugars become concentrated and the flavors intensify. You don't have to add any sugar or fat. You can dehydrate all kinds of produce such as bananas, cherries, tomatoes, apples, plums, and apricots.

In order to safely dehydrate food, you need dry, controlled heat to force moisture from the food, and air circulation to carry the moisture away.

When food is dehydrated, 80 to 95 percent of the moisture is removed, so bacteria and other spoilage microorganisms can't grow. But drying doesn't kill the microorganisms already present. The food can still spoil if not enough moisture is removed.

An electric dehydrator provides the most reliable and consistent results for drying foods because of the controlled temperature and airflow.

You can also dry food outdoors, but you need bright, hot sunshine; low humidity; and low air pollution. The *Ball Blue Book Guide to Preserving* advises daytime temperatures of at least 90 degrees. The hotter the weather, the faster, and more safely, your foods will dry. Also, you need a screen or netting to protect the food from insects.

If you have a dehydrator, follow your manufacturer's instructions for best results. It's a simple, straightforward process: Wash, peel, and pit the produce; cut or slice in uniform pieces. Dip fruits such as apples, bananas, and peaches in pineapple or lemon juice to keep them from oxidizing and turning brown. Then place them on the dehydrator screen. Cover with the lid and turn the dehydrator on. Dry until crisp and moisture is removed.

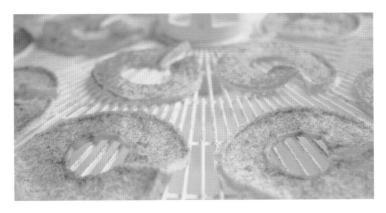

Dried Apple Chips

My neighbor Sharon Hansen dries apples for Tagge's fruit stands. Last year she gave me some for the holidays. I asked her to show me how to make these delicious apple chips, and she did. I now have a new skill.

Here is what you will need to make apple chips:

A dehydrator, apple peeler (it peels, cores, and slices all in one process), 1 large can pineapple juice, waxed paper or plastic wrap, a knife, and lots of apples. The dehydrator that I used had 10 trays.

The first step is to wash the apples and set up the apple peeler. Spread waxed paper or plastic wrap on the counter and pour the pineapple juice into a bowl. Set up your work station so you can peel the apples, dip them in pineapple juice, and place them right on the dehydrator trays.

Place the stem end of an apple into the three prongs of the peeler arm. Turn until the apple is peeled, sliced, and cored. Set the apple on the tray, and with the paring knife cut a slit in the apple all the way to the bottom. Now place the apple slices into the pineapple juice, making sure all slices are covered, as this will keep them from darkening. Put the individual slices onto the de-hydrator tray. As you fill a tray, place it on the dehydrator.

Once all the trays are filled and in place, turn the dehydrator on. My dehydrator takes 6 or 7 hours to dry apples. At 3 hours, I open the dehydrator and turn the apples over tray by tray. This keeps them from sticking to the trays once dried.

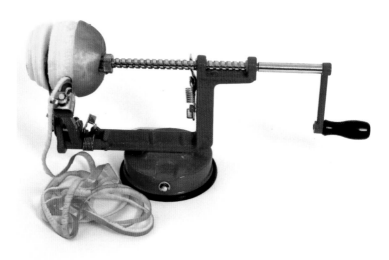

Question: What are some of your favorite recipes that would help you achieve your weight-loss goals?

_____

_____

_____

_____

_____

_____

_____

_____

_____

_____

_____

_____

_____

_____

_____

_____

_____

_____

_____

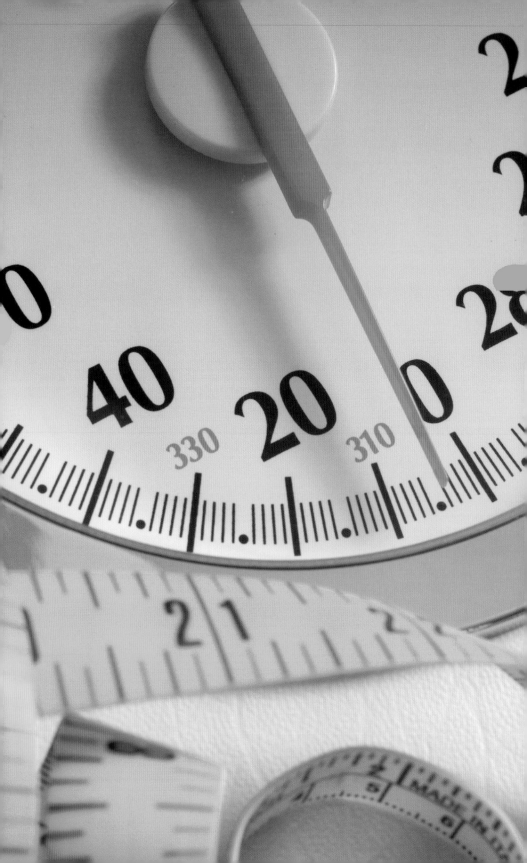

Chapter 9
Willpower or Willingness?

Dieters know how much willpower it takes to follow their regimens. The real challenge of a diet is—how hard it is to keep it up for the rest of your life. Sooner or later, most people go back to eating as they used to, often putting on more weight than they lost. I finally decided I was through with that.

Jackie Keller showed me a different way. Her program was not based on willpower but willingness to do what it took to change my lifestyle. Small steps allowed me to become successful at losing weight over a period of time, each step building on the previous success. Patience was key in this process.

Jackie helped me set up a program not dependent on willpower. Here are my six "willingness" steps.

1. Willingness to set up my home environment for success. The first thing I did was give away the unhealthy foods. Then I worked hard to ban from my home things that required great willpower to resist. If this is a hardship for your family, perhaps you can ask them to keep tempting foods out of sight.

2. Willingness to shop once a week for nutritious foods. No picking up an item at the store because it looked good or that I was suddenly in the mood for, unless it fit into my designated meal plan.

3. Willingness to take time to prepare my food in advance so it is organized and accessible when I'm ready to eat. None of my meals take more than fifteen minutes to prepare.

4. Willingness to be active every day.

    a.   I wear a pedometer and strive for 10,000 to 12,000 steps each day. I take work breaks and time at lunch to do a little walking, and walk whenever I can enjoy a sunset or sunrise.

    b.   I worked with a trainer who developed a routine that would strengthen me.

    c.   I found an activity (bike riding) that I love. It has become part of my lifestyle.

    d.   I look for opportunities to work in functional exercise, such as planting a garden, mowing the lawn, shoveling snow, painting the walls, and cleaning the house.

5. Willingness to eat three meals and three snacks a day to keep my metabolism at full steam.

6. Willingness to add vegetables as a major part of my diet.

    a.   Each day I strive to include a variety of vegetables—two to three for both lunch and dinner.

    b.   I eat fresh or frozen vegetables—I avoid commercially processed vegetables.

Small adjustments can make a big difference in your health, your weight, and your happiness. When you put plenty of "willingness" into developing a program that supports weight loss and stay with it, you will find the weight will come off—and stay off!

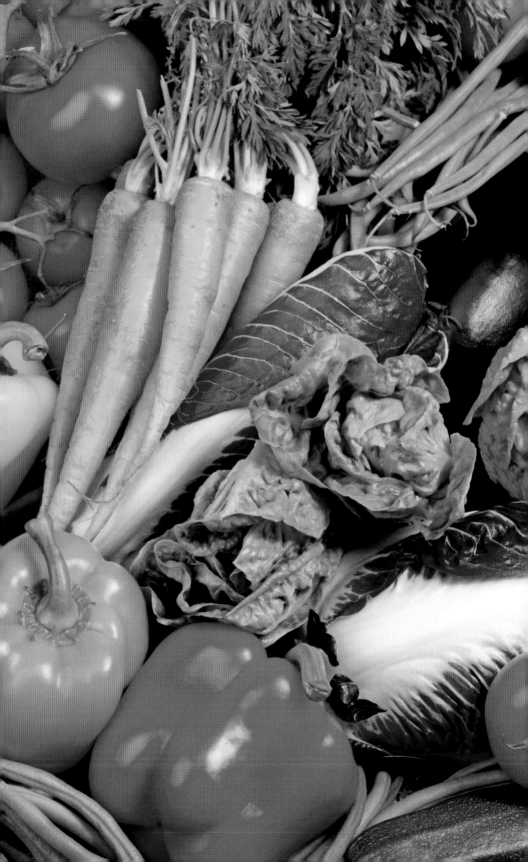

Appendix

MARKET ORDER

PRODUCE	DAIRY	MEAT

FROZEN	CANNED	DRY GOODS

HOUSEHOLD SUPPLIES	MISC.	OTHER ERRANDS

Index

Stock soup, 157
Strategies, 2, 32, 87, 95–98,
Strength training, 47–48, 111,
134
Stroke, 79
Sugar alcohols, 73
Surgeon General, 44, 134
Swimming, 4, 12, 36–37,
39, 51

T

Tai Chi, 37, 63
Television, 6–7, 15, 33,
88, 133
Temptation, 80, 94
Thai, 120, 122, 166
Thailand, 13, 28
Three P's in a Pod, 22–27
Thyme, 121, 152, 160–161,
166
Tomato sauce, 110, 143, 150–
151, 187, 196–197
Tracy, Brian, 23
Trans fats, 69, 72, 74
Travolta, John, 51
Turmeric, 120
Turkey burgers, 120, 179
Turkey stock, 160

U

Ultra Gel, 101
University of North Carolina
Nutrition Obesity, 82
University of Tennessee, 43
University of Utah, 80
USDA, 67, 72–73, 82, 89, 91,
113, 127, 135, 171, 196
USDA's Extension Services,
196

V

Vegetable stock, 161
Vegetables for sandwiches,
175

Vegetables for soups, 162
Vietnamese, 120
Virginia Tech, 81
Vitamins, 68–69, 74, 85, 125,
127–128

W

Walking, 1, 4, 9, 35, 38–39,
42–44, 48–50, 53, 57, 204
Walking salad, 172
Waltman, Floss, 9
Ward, William Arthur, 24
Warm-up, 111
Water aerobics, 1, 4, 12,
38–39, 111
Web sites, 113, 154
Weight Watchers Scale, 104
Wii, 52
Willingness, 203–204
Willpower, 203
Wraps, 174–177

Y

Yard work, 50

Z

Ziploc sandwich bags, 90, 94,
100, 104, 193

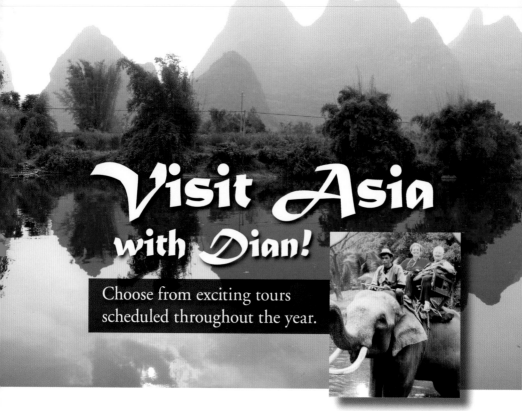

Visit Asia with Dian!

Choose from exciting tours scheduled throughout the year.

You can travel to China or Thailand with Dian Thomas as your guide! As a frequent visitor to Asia, Dian has become an expert and can show you why she loves the people and places so much.

With Dian as your guide, you'll experience the culture and cuisine and visit the legendary sites of the Orient. But most importantly,

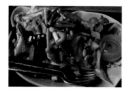

you'll really get to know the people of China and Thailand and make connections that will change your life *for the better*.

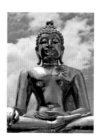

Highlights of the China tour include hiking the Great Wall of China, exploring the Forbidden City, visiting Beijing's Olympic sites, and shopping at designer clothing markets. You and your family and friends won't forget this *magical* tour.

For more information, go to: www.DianThomas.com/travel.htm
or e-mail travel@DianThomas.com.

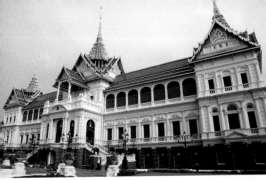
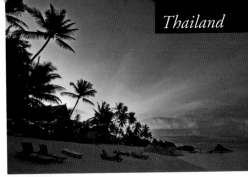

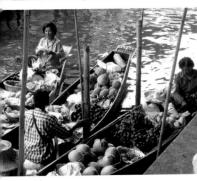
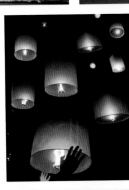
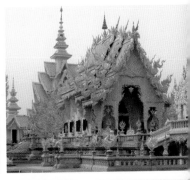

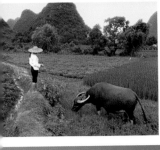
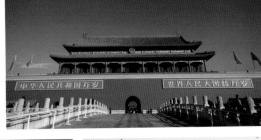
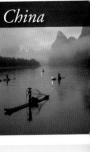

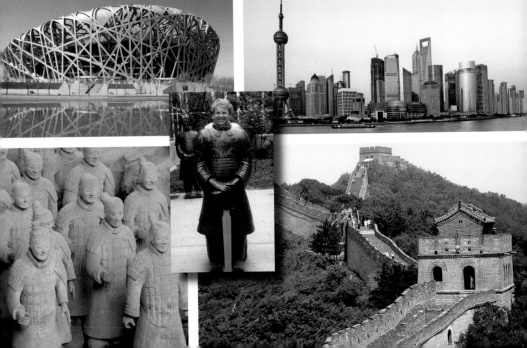

There's more *fun* from Dian!

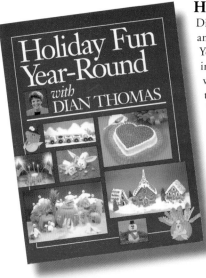

Holiday Fun Year-Round

Dian Thomas's collection of festive ideas and recipes will make every holiday special. You'll discover interesting tidbits of information about many holidays, why we observe them, and how to celebrate them with fun.

You'll discover ideas for:

- A super Super Bowl party
- An exciting egg hunt for Easter
- Homemade gifts for Mother's Day and Father's Day
- Eerie decorations, creative costumes, and spooky treats for Halloween
- Creative Christmas ideas . . . and more.

From New Year's to Christmas.
182 pages, full-color photos. $19.99

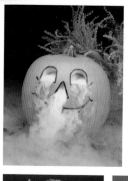
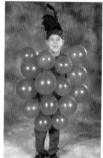
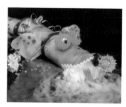
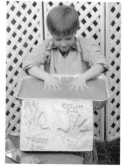
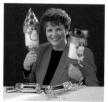
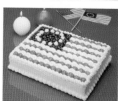

For more information and to order, visit Dian's
Web site: www.DianThomas.com/products.htm

Recipes for Roughing It Easy

Novices will appreciate Dian's tips on packing food for camping, creating a portable pantry, preparing scrumptious meals, or making intended leftovers. Experienced campers will relish Dian's favorite ideas for novelty cooking—such as cooking chicken in a backpack while hiking, frying eggs and bacon in a paper bag, and even making ice cream in the woods! *240 pages. $14.99*

 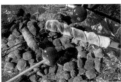 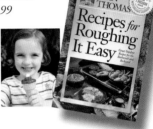

Backyard Roughing It Easy

Dian answers all of your questions from how to start a fire to the do's and don'ts of planning a backyard camping trip with your family. Don't have a grill? Why not turn an ash can into a newspaper stove? Need tips for easy outdoor entertaining? Look no further; Dian's recipes and party ideas will make you the talk of the town. You'll never look at your backyard the same way again. *180 pages. $14.99*

  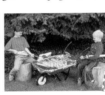 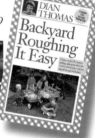

Roughing It Easy

This *New York Times* best-seller is chock-full of recipes and great ideas. Cook eggs and bacon in a paper bag, and start a fire with steel wool and batteries! Expert advice for equipment selection, fire building, campfire cooking, solar cooking, and drying your own foods for backpacking! This new, expanded edition also includes emergency planning for home, family, and auto. *272 pages. $14.99*

  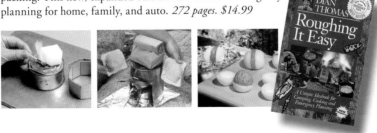

For more information and to order, visit Dian's
Web site: www.DianThomas.com/products.htm
